BONDAGE
Basics

Naughty Knots
and Risqué Restraints
You Need to Know

BONDAGE
Basics

LORD MORPHEOUS

Foreword by Jessica O'Reilly, Ph.D.,
author of *The Little Book of Kink*

QUIVER

Quarto.com

© 2015 Quiver
Text and Photography © 2015 Quiver

First published in 2015 by Quiver,
an imprint of The Quarto Group,
100 Cummings Center, Suite 265-D,
Beverly, MA 01915, USA.
T (978) 282-9590 F (978) 283-2742

Quiver titles are also available at discount for retail, wholesale, promotional, and bulk purchase. For details, contact the Special Sales Manager by email at specialsales@quarto.com or by mail at The Quarto Group, Attn: Special Sales Manager, 100 Cummings Center, Suite 265-D, Beverly, MA 01915, USA.

The Publisher maintains the records relating to images in this book required by 18 USC 2257. Records are located at Rockport Publishers, Inc., 100 Cummings Center, Suite 406-L, Beverly, MA 01915-6101.

26 25 24 23   9 10 11 12 13

ISBN: 978-1-59233-645-6

Digital edition published in 2015
eISBN: 978-1-62788-189-0

Library of Congress Cataloging-in-Publication Data available

Cover design by Sporto
Book design by Sporto
Photography by Holly Randall, except as follows:
Morpheous, pages 24, 28, 30, 43, 72, 76, 82, 158, and 160
Geoff George Photography, pages 49, 54, 56, 57, 58, 60, 63, 64, 65, 84, 86-99, 106, and 107
Front cover photo by Lord Morpheous, rigged by Ruairidh, model: Kerry Maguire

Printed and bound in Hong Kong

To everyone who has ever been involved in MBE, and most of all
to Princess and My Allyss, who have always believed in me . . .
and to the OLG.

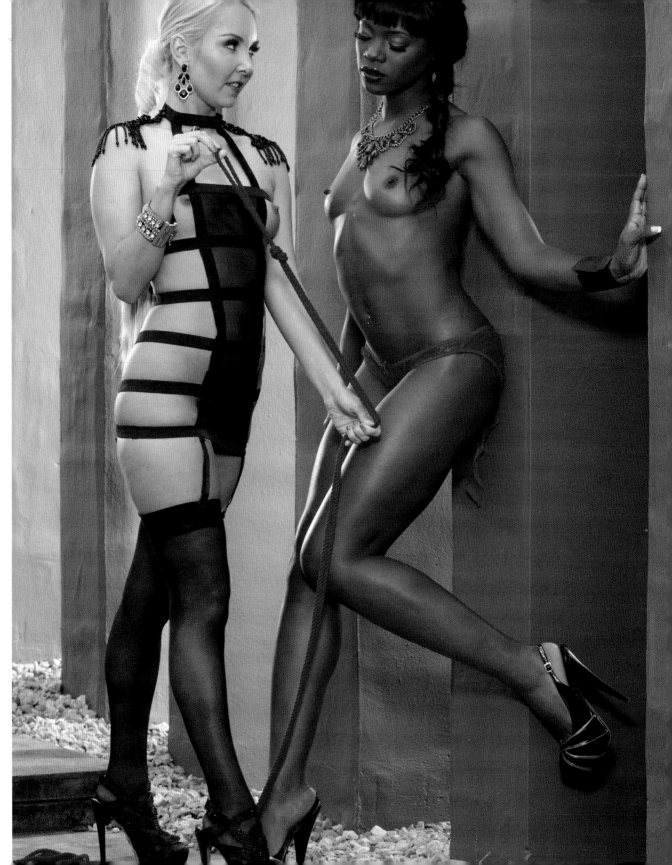

Contents

Foreword

I first met Morpheous a few years back at his local breakfast haunt in Toronto. As he approached, clad in all black from head to toe, I felt a powerful presence descend upon me. I'm unsure if it was his height, his saunter, or simply his energy, but there was something undeniably and unsurprisingly *dominant* about the way he carried himself. When he reached out to shake my hand and introduce himself with a smile, however, his decided strength was immediately overshadowed by his warmth and mild-mannered nature. It took only a short moment for me to appreciate that beneath the ostensibly intense exterior was a man of complexity, humility, and kindness.

Bondage Basics reflects this complexity of character, offering a balance of humor, playfulness, education, sensuality, eroticism, and practical advice for beginner and intermediate rope play. Morpheous brilliantly weaves personal anecdotes together with standard best practices to offer a thorough exploration of bondage as a form of art and pleasure. From the onset, it is apparent that the author has put great personal care into the text in the same fashion as he would when playing out a scene with one of his rope bunnies.

When I first opened this book, I was struck by the beautiful images and was surprised to see a few familiar faces . . . and rear ends! Morpheous clearly had a hand in selecting the models and styling the shoot. And though the aesthetic appeal of *Bondage Basics* is indisputable, it is the text that is most meaningful, thoughtful, and moving. Reading this book, I couldn't help but develop a more profound appreciation for rope play and its expressive bond with BDSM. While I have always loved being tied up and have long considered power play (see page 83) the most delightful of all sexual indulgences, I was admittedly a rope play neophyte before sinking my teeth into Morpheous' latest book. Upon completion of the text, not only have I been inspired to replace my silk scarves and designer neckties with a selection of soft, pink nylon rope, but the author's review of the fascinating history associated with this "loving, sensual, and erotic activity" has broadened my perception of rope bondage in terms of art, pleasure, and cultural practice.

The public's interest in kink has also broadened over the last few years with the rise of BDSM-themed books and movies. And while these fictional stories have sparked an important dialogue about consent, relationships, and kinky sex play, those fictional accounts offer little to no direction with regard to the implementation of kink. That's where *Bondage Basics* comes in.

Though I had read and studied hundreds of sexuality books before reviewing *Bondage Basics*, I still learned a great deal from Morpheous' new material. From reviewing standard terminology and offering sage advice for effective communication, to providing step-by-step introductions for knot tying and negotiating boundaries, *Bondage Basics* guides the reader on an exciting and kinky journey. Each chapter builds upon the former in a natural and easy-to-follow sequence. And because the risk associated with rope play may be higher than other forms sexual activity, the author complements every move, technique, and strategy with sensible safety advice, which is sure to be relevant to newbie and experienced kinksters alike.

In addition to offering a more expansive perspective on bondage, Morpheous, who is renowned for valuing and protecting his personal privacy, also offers readers a rare glimpse into his personal story. I'm not the least bit surprised to learn that he grew up on a farm—he certainly doesn't mind getting his hands more than a little dirty—and I'm equally unsurprised to discover that the world's largest bondage event, which he launched over a decade ago, is free to attend, as he has a reputation for his generosity of spirit, time, and resources. The author's passion for bondage may have made him an involuntary innovator in his early years of experimentation, but *Bondage Basics* will ensure that Morpheous' cultural influence endures as readers are inspired to carve out their own paths and develop their own meaningful innovations.

Morpheous is not just a kink educator and sought-after expert; he's also a collector, connoisseur, and trailblazer in the field of rope bondage and BDSM. It is an honor and pleasure to both preview and offer a small contribution to such an important and beautiful project.

Read with pleasure!

—**Jessica O'Reilly, Ph.D.**
Author of *The Little Book of Kink* and *The New Sex Bible*
www.SexWithDrJess.com

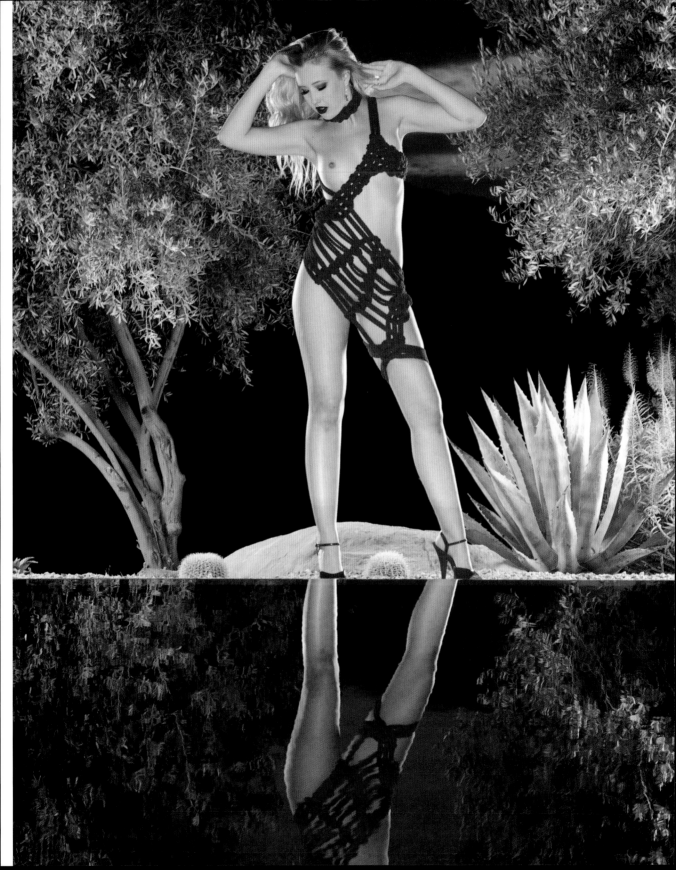

ALL ABOUT KINK

Regardless of what they'd like you to believe, absolutely everyone has a kink.

When we first begin to explore the more kinky sides of our sexual personalities, it can feel scary, as if we're catapulting ourselves into a world that we don't understand. The aim of this book is not to tell you what you should like. The aim of this book is to help you explore your sexuality and artistic abilities and to imbue you with rope bondage skills to take your new hobby and grow with it.

I grew up on a farm where using rope was a practical, day-to-day skill. Different knots perform different duties. I learned the right ones for the job from my grandfather. Eventually, I wound up in a relationship with a kinky girl who wanted to be tied up. So one night, I tied her up the only way I knew how—like a wagonload of hay. We laughed about it, but she couldn't get out of it. None of her other lovers had ever tied her up like that before, to a point where she couldn't escape, and, to my delight, it turned her on immensely! We explored and experienced the pleasures of rope bondage with each other for a few years, and then the Internet happened.

In those days, my friends and I would stumble across Japanese websites depicting women tied in luscious ways. But none of us could read Japanese, so we did the only thing we could do: We tried to reverse engineer the ties. Clearly, this posed a huge challenge. Though we never perfected the ties, we ended up bringing our own skills to the table and were problem solving with our Western skill set and approach to bondage.

Around this time, I discovered Lew Rubens (who would later become a close friend and terrific inspiration) online and was amazed at the work he was creating. Thankfully, his work was in English. That made practicing rope techniques much easier, especially with the approach Lew took, inspired by long-ago Western bondage masters like John Willie. I learned the beauty of making bondage simple and utilitarian, leaving room for inspiration and flourishes.

Eventually, I would meet another great friend, Midori, who would give me some hands-on training in Japanese-style bondage. She always maintained that the work could never be "truly Japanese," because there were differences in the way she tied and what was taking place in Japan. Nevertheless, it was a great opportunity to have more detailed instruction in Eastern knot tying.

I would eventually become inspired by Arisue Go and Osada Steve and the work I saw in Japanese books. However, I never strayed far from my Western roots and incorporated as much of my own style into what I was seeing and practicing. One of the most satisfying aspects was to work out problems with knots in my own style with the skills I had developed.

I remember when the rope bondage scene in Toronto was exactly three people—my two friends and me. But our rope masterpieces inspired others at fetish nights to practice their own forms of rope bondage. The love of rope bondage in the fetish community became so strong that it needed a larger audience. That passion is what drove me to create and host the world's largest public rope bondage event called Morpheous' Bondage Extravaganza (MBE). The event takes place in Toronto annually in October and is approaching its tenth year. It is free to the public and showcases the best rope bondage artists around the world for one sleepless night, from sundown to sunrise. The event is now on the international spectrum and takes place concurrently in different cities around the world.

These days, I draw my inspiration from great works of art and from nature. The range of human emotions and expression has been conveyed through countless works of art over the ages. From postimpressionist painting to renaissance sculpture to postmodernity and photography, I look at other artists' approaches and inspiration to motivate my own art. I want to thank the team I put together of the best rope artists I know (Allura, Ruairidh, and Ve-ra) who helped me rig, style, and bring this book to you.

We all come to rope bondage in different ways, and our paths through it will be equally different. Perhaps you've felt the soft tug of rope against your fleshy bits while playing with a partner who was into bondage. Perhaps you accidently walked into a rope bondage exhibition once and felt a stirring in a place that you've never felt before. Perhaps you saw this book in a store and picked it up on impulse because the cover attracted you for some reason you can't pinpoint. No matter how you arrived here, I hope that this book will be the first step on a journey that takes you wherever you want to go—and beyond where you think you might end up, all while having fun and playing safely.

Now sit back, relax, and get ready to be tantalized.

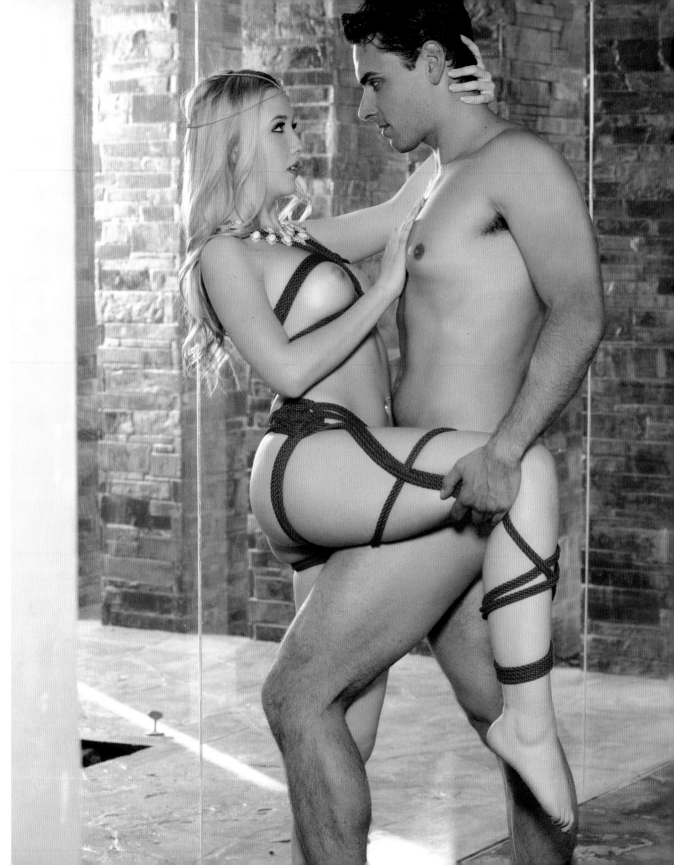

Chapter 1

BONDAGE 101

If you've picked up this book, I'm going to assume that you're interested in bringing a little more kink into your life—either that, or someone bought you a wildly inappropriate Secret Santa gift. In the case of the former: Excellent! Welcome to your first step into a world of writhing bodies, excited panting, and getting a hell of a lot filthier than you originally thought you were.

Rope bondage, for me, is the most loving, sensual, and erotic activity that you and a partner (or two, or three) can engage in. I love the feel of rope running through my hands as I truss up a submissive in a harness tie, her skin becoming warmer under my hands as her excitement grows. I love the smell of rope after a session, and the sound of nylon running over metal as you suspend your partner. I love the way that rope bondage is an agreement of trust as well as of passion, and the way that it brings a couple closer together by putting love and care at the forefront of every scene. To me, rope bondage is simply the best way that you can spend an evening (or late afternoon, or morning), and I'm thrilled that you're coming on this journey into beginner's rope bondage with me.

But first, the basics: Bondage is the practice of tying or restraining a partner for sexual or artistic purposes. In this book we'll be talking mostly about bondage with rope, simply because it is the most fun. Bondage is often discussed in the wider category of BDSM, as it tends to overlap with other kinky activities (and is all the better for it, if you ask me), some of which you'll find yourself interested in and some of which you won't. That's totally fine; your journey through rope bondage is your own, and you should find your own path.

Now, if the kinkiest thing you've ever done in the bedroom is leave the door open when the kids were due home, the term "BDSM" can seem a little intimidating. Popular culture and books and movies that feature BDSM relationships have also left a lot of people thinking that these relationhips must be abusive. This is far, far from the truth. The BDSM community values trust, safety, and communication above all else and engages in pain for pleasure only in a consensual and loving setting. Even if BDSM is a fairly new concept to you, you've probably already strayed a lot closer to BDSM-style sexual expression than you think; whether it was using those pink, fluffy handcuffs someone bought you for your twenty-first birthday or accidentally whipping your partner while you were trying to seductively remove his belt that one time, the chances are you've experienced a little bit of pain for pleasure at least once in your life. If not, don't worry. That's what this book is for.

Let's start from the very beginning. What does BDSM mean?

BDSM isn't one specific acronym. Instead, it takes in the three concepts of bondage and discipline, dominance and submission, and sadism and masochism. Named after the Marquis de Sade, the eighteenth-century French aristocrat who was imprisoned for writing salacious erotic literature that focused on pain and pleasure, sadism is the experience of pleasure through inflicting pain, while masochism is the experience of pleasure while receiving pain. These terms have been used over the years to describe these experiences as paraphilia (or "strange" sexual practices), especially in medical texts, so most of us in the various BDSM communities prefer the term "sadomasochist" these days. This also describes the fluid sexuality that can allow people to enjoy being both dominant and submissive, or both giving and receiving pleasure through pain—although doing both at the same time can cause chafing and a bad back.

If all this seems too much like the movie *Secretary*, don't be alarmed (unless you loved that movie, in which case, it's exactly like that). BDSM activities range in intensity, and almost anything, when done right, can come under the BDSM umbrella. Tying your husband's wrists to the bedframe with his neckties and making him watch you do a striptease is BDSM; so is buying your first 6-inch strap-on and making him beg you to use it on him. There are a million and one different ways to enjoy BDSM and you should never feel pressured to go beyond your own personal boundaries—although exploring where exactly your boundaries lie is part of the fun!

In this book, however, we're going to focus on the bondage and discipline part of BDSM, and more specifically on the bondage element. This includes bondage using rope and bondage using classic items that are found around the house or on your person, like scarves, belts, and men's ties. I am going to show you how to make it safe and sexy at the same time. If you feel like the other BDSM stuff sounds better than a night in watching reality TV and eating cold mac 'n' cheese, then you can find many useful links and book titles at the back of this book under the resources section (and remember—your best friend is your dirty mind!). This chapter serves as a fluffer, if you will, before we get to the main event: the rope!

VOCABULARY

Like every subculture, BDSM has its terms, phrases, and jargon. Here's a short list of some of the most important terms to learn when you're starting, but you'll no doubt pick up a lot more along your journey. Just don't repeat any of these in front of your mother.

aftercare: The physical and mental support given to a submissive by the dominant partner(s) after BDSM play.

bondage: The practice of tying or restraining a person, most commonly so that they are immobile. A whole host of materials can be used, but rope is the most common and most popular.

bottom: A person who plays a submissive role when required. A bottom may not naturally be a submissive, but may take the role in a particular scene if no other submissive is present.

collaring: To engage in a committed, long-term dominant-submissive relationship. The dominant may place a collar upon the submissive during a special ceremony.

consent: The most important concept in all of BDSM, this is affirmative permission, given in sound mind. RACK (risk-aware consensual kink) is a code of conduct in the BDSM community and it is very much adhered to.

daddy: A person who takes on the role of a dominant to one or more submissives. This role is nurturing and loving, and may involve education and emotional support as well as general dominant activities.

dominant (or dom): A person who likes to be sexually dominant and takes on a role of power or authority over submissives in a power exchange. The dominant is generally in control of a scene with others and calls the shots.

domme: A female dominant, or a professional dominatrix. A domme may provide nonsexual dominance services to clients.

hard limits: The lines over which a person will not cross, and which they do not want to approach too closely.

master/mistress: A person who lives the BDSM lifestyle 24/7 and has committed to dominating a slave in a total power exchange (TPE).

rigger: A universal term for someone who likes to tie up others. Closely associated with the next term.

rope bunny: A person, of any gender, who gets hot and bothered being tied up or restrained by rope. Bunnies aren't necessarily submissive by nature, but they love a good rope burn as much as the next masochist.

safe word: The code word that a submissive can use whenever play becomes too much. A safe word stops all play immediately, and its use is nonnegotiable. A safe word is particularly important in scenes where resistance play is expected; for instance, when a submissive may say no as part of the play. I recommend using "green," "yellow," and "red"—just like a stoplight.

scene: A session of BDSM play. "Scene" can also be used to refer to the BDSM community as a whole.

sensation play: A type of BDSM activity that plays with a submissive's sensations. For instance, this may involve hot wax, ice, abrasive materials, and fur. This may or may not escalate into pain play.

slave: A person who lives the BDSM lifestyle 24/7 and has committed to being under his or her master's control entirely. This is the other role in a TPE.

soft limits: The boundaries over which a person may cross, if the situation is right. Soft limits are fun to explore, but a person should never be coerced into going beyond what he or she is comfortable with.

submissive (or sub): A person who assumes a more submissive, passive role in a power exchange. Although this is usually sexual, some submissives are service-oriented, in that they seek to serve a master or mistress in a practical way without any overt sexual power exchange.

subdrop: The "low" feeling that a submissive may experience after a particularly intense scene or play session. Although correct aftercare can mitigate these feelings, the "down" state can last for hours or even days.

subspace: The dreamy, euphoric state into which submissives can fall during a particularly intense scene or play session. In subspace, the rest of the world seems to fall away, and the feeling of bliss can last for hours or even days afterward.

switch: A person who switches between top and bottom roles whenever they feel like it. These are the most fun people to play with, as they can move between the two roles according to need and desire.

top: A person who plays a dominant role when required. A top may only play as top for the enjoyment of his or her master, for instance, and may be more naturally a submissive.

total power exchange (TPE): A relationship in which one person (the slave) voluntarily and consensually gives another (the master/mistress) total control and authority over him or her. This is generally a 24/7 agreement and may be open-ended, or may last for a finite time.

FINDING YOUR ROLE

When you're first beginning to explore your kinky side, it can be difficult to know just what type of role will fit you best, or whether in fact you're one of those lucky devils that will get just as hot wielding a whip as you will be on the receiving end of those tasty lashes. You might get a kick out being spanked on occasion, but will you love being hogtied and played with, only allowed to cum when your mistress tells you to? You might love to tie your partner's arms and legs to the bed to play with him or her, but are you ready for the responsibility of someone else giving himself or herself up to you totally?

It's important to remember that there are a multitude of roles in BDSM and that the whole spectrum of human sexuality can never be boiled down to just one or two narrow categories. That said, some people find great comfort in moving from one role to another, as the boundaries therein can help them explore all possible experiences. A sub one day might suddenly feel that he or she is ready for a 24/7 slave role and might flourish under strict orders from his or her master. No one can ever tell you which role is right for you; rather, the way to find your role is to experiment, keep an open mind, and try each one on. Like a good dress or a suit, you'll likely know which one suits you perfectly as soon as you try it on, but you may need to try a few different styles on in the beginning.

You might still have questions after your first, second, fourth, tenth, or twentieth play session. That's okay; some people never feel comfortable putting labels on themselves and instead prefer to exist in the fluid, fluctuating space of sexuality that BDSM easily allows. BDSM is a journey, and if you never quite find a destination, you're still in for a hell of a lot of fun.

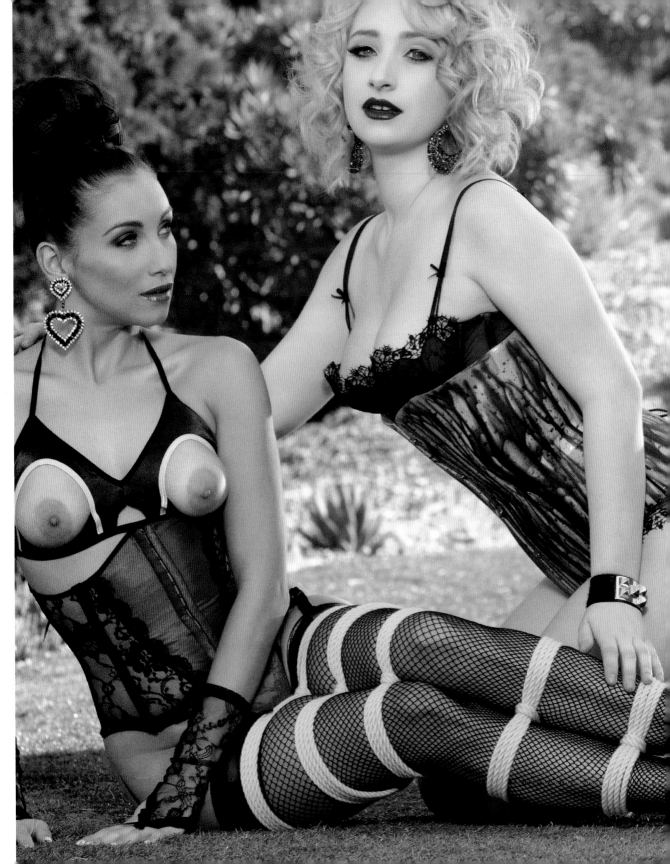

AFTERCARE

They say that what goes up must come down, and this is especially true in the world of BDSM. During play, the submissives in a scene sometimes reach a state known as subspace, in which all cares and troubles, and even pain, fall away and the sub exists in a dream state of euphoria. In this way, it isn't completely dissimilar to being drunk or high on drugs, and the feelings after this sensation subsides can also be the same as those coming off drugs.

The phenomenon of coming down after a scene is known as subdrop. This is caused by those delicious endorphins leaving your body and sending you into withdrawal. The intensity of this "down" feeling can range from a few hours of feeling sad and physically exhausted to a week feeling numb and a little lost. For most people, especially when dealing with the sort of bondage in this book, the down feeling might simply be a sense of vulnerability. However, it's important that everyone leaves a scene feeling cared for and nurtured, and for this reason, it's incredibly important that any play session, even light bondage, involves a good amount of aftercare for all involved. In fact, you should be sure to discuss aftercare in your negotiation process with any new partner. The negotiation process is the period before play begins, in which you lay down all ground rules and boundaries, talk about any health issues that may affect play, and generally ensure that all parties are comfortable. Aftercare is as necessary as foreplay in the BDSM world—and can be just as erotic too.

The physical effects of a scene, especially a rope bondage scene, can be obvious; cuts, bruises, and abrasions should be taken care of as quickly as possible, with any cuts being sterilized and bandaged, and creams such as Arnica applied to bruising to help with recovery. Think of this as the "doctor and nurses" portion of the evening, and it will become a lot more fun. Drink something sweet and have lots of water, and if you're hungry, eat something carby and healthy. It goes without saying that if you have sustained any serious injuries, or any of your bruises seem more intense than normal, you should seek medical attention immediately.

◄ *Are you ready for someone to give him- or herself up to you totally?*

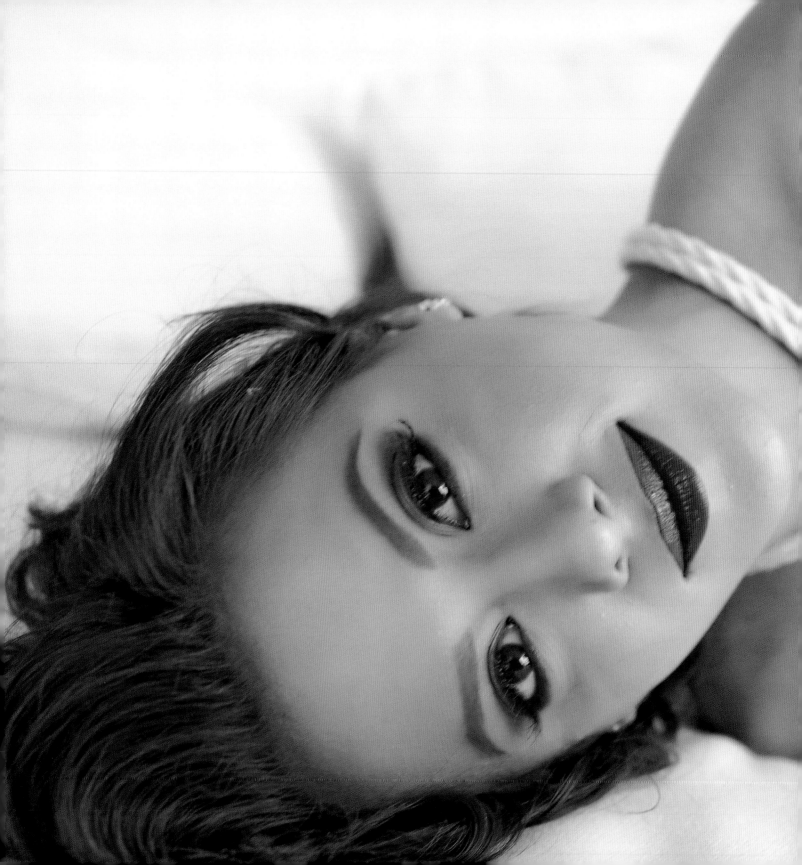

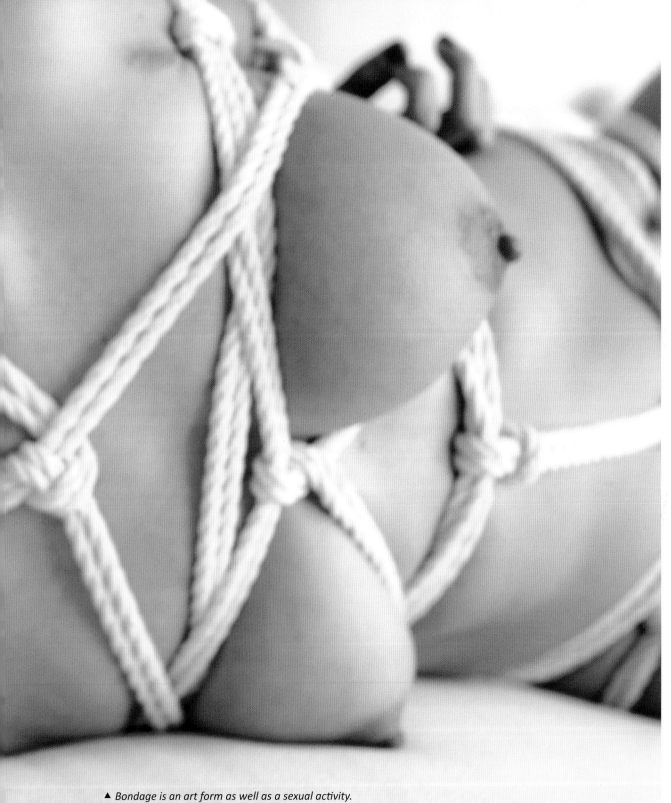

▲ Bondage is an art form as well as a sexual activity.

Emotional aftercare can take many forms, but the dominant in the scene should take care to ensure that the space is a comforting and relaxing one, and should also address any feelings that the sub(s) express, as well as providing positive reinforcement, which can be as simple as "you're a good little thing, yes, you are." Soft physical contact can be reassuring for some people, and good-quality dark chocolate can actually help with subdrop, which is surely as good an excuse as any to indulge in a little treat after play.

Sometimes it's necessary to provide yourself with aftercare, if your play partners aren't available after the scene or if you just decide that you'd prefer to be alone. It's good to have a little "aftercare pack" for yourself, so you can make yourself comfortable and deal with feelings that you think may arise. Include something that makes you feel good about yourself, whether that's a letter from a lover or an email from a friend, and include body cream, a DVD of your favorite movie, relaxing music, candles, incense, and candies to make sure you can create a comforting environment. Always make sure you have a phone to call someone if you're feeling lonely—and don't forget the chocolate.

ROPE BONDAGE AND BDSM

Now we get to the part that I really love—the bondage. Bondage in BDSM refers to the practice of tying up or restraining a partner/partners for sexual activity, decoration, power play, or art. When you use old stockings with a run in them to tie your boyfriend's hands behind his back so that he can't touch you while you're teasing him, that's bondage. When you find yourself bound to a bedframe, unable to twist your wrists without the duct tape pressing into your vulnerable flesh, that's bondage. When a submissive gets into a vacuum bed and has all the air slowly sucked out, leaving the latex layers with nothing to do other than cling to his or her sensuous curves, which beg to be played with, that's bondage.

Bondage, in many forms, already plays a role in many people's sex lives, but in BDSM, bondage becomes a central part of playtime for many. Some of us love nothing more than to spend our evenings tying up our partners, and we affectionately call them "rope bunnies" in the scene, regardless of their gender. Though others may not get wet thinking about being hogtied and flogged, they might enjoy toe cuffs, having their fingers, hands, feet, or bodies tied up with colored wool, or lots of other fun bondage play with rope. Although many materials can be used to restrict or tie someone, rope is the preferred material of many (including me), thanks to its resilience, ease of use, and versatility. It's a sex toy that doesn't require batteries, doesn't require a lot of preparation time, doesn't get your fingers all covered in lube, and doesn't shock your family if it is sitting in a drawer and they stumble across it looking for stamps (will they believe you're a rock climber?). There are many different types of rope, and I am going to show a variety in this book, but if you are starting out, soft nylon rope is a cheap and easy type to use because it is strong, fun to work with, and soft and supple on your sub's vulnerable, precious skin.

Bondage can be an art form as well as a method by which to have your filthy way with your submissive, and not all rope bondage is engaged in for sexual reasons. In fact, rope as an art form has a long history. My annual rope bondage display, Morpheous' Bondage Extravaganza, is a twelve-hour showcase of the beauty and art inherent in rope, and its huge attendance and online viewership just goes to show that rope can be gorgeous even to those outside of the scene. In BDSM, though, rope is often used in scenes to restrict a submissive's movements for stimulation and play, and can also serve as a great way to keep your partner in that sexy-as-hell position while you ravish him or her senseless. There are many ways in which bondage can be used in BDSM that's neither sexual nor artistic; for instance, finger or toe bondage can keep your service-oriented slave in the correct mind-set to serve you, and a crude rope chastity belt can remind your submissive who she belongs to while she's at work. Some bunnies love the feel of rough jute rope against their skin while they're teased and tickled; others enjoy soft hemp or cotton rope, and still others love the act of being tied and enjoy the headspace that bondage puts them into, without needing any extra stimulation. There is no right way to incorporate bondage into your life, and finding out what floats your boat is half the fun!

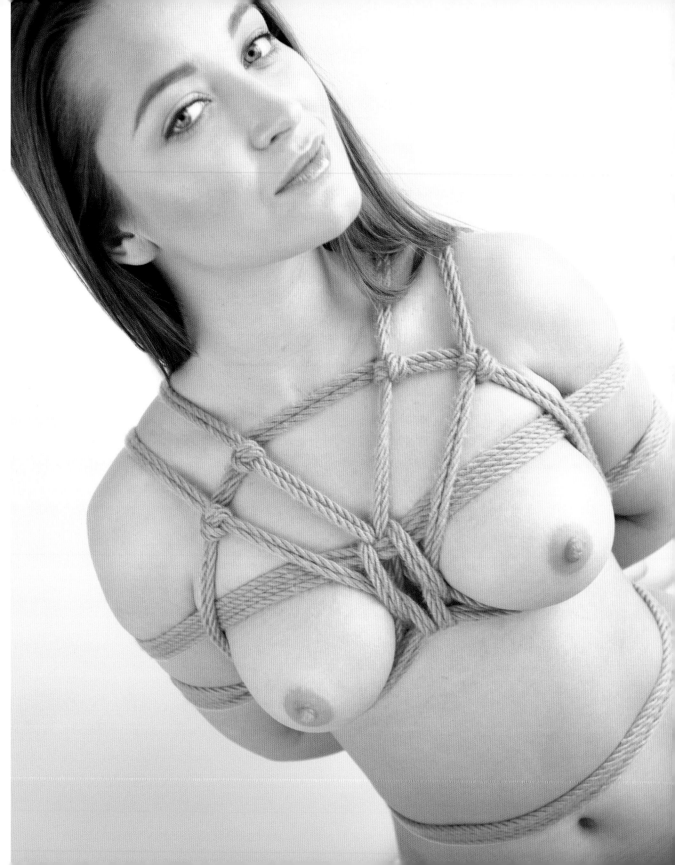

Chapter 2

THE HISTORY OF
ROPE BONDAGE

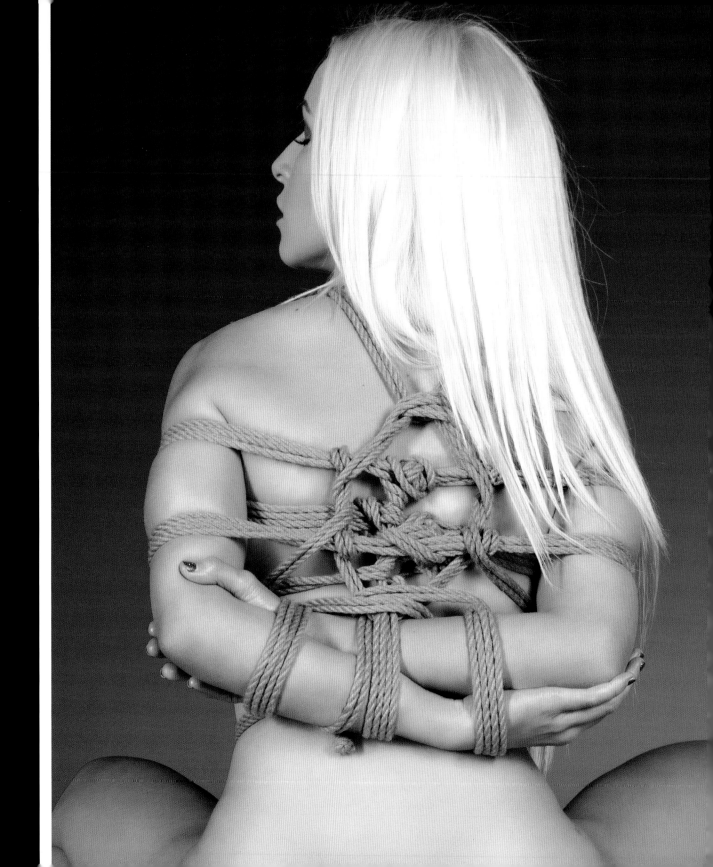

EASTERN ROPE BONDAGE

The Eastern school of rope bondage has an incredibly long history, although it is generally accepted that it has its roots in the Japanese practice of *hojōjutsu*, a martial art of restraining people using rope or sometimes cord. Related to both *budō* and *jujitsu*, *hojōjutsu* was practiced by the samurai (those kinky devils) as one of the eighteen essential fighting arts and is part of a greater cultural practice of tying that goes back over a millennium, but it's difficult to pinpoint when *hojōjutsu* was first used. What we can be sure of, however, is that its use grew exponentially from 1600 onward before more specific offshoots of tying and restraining began to appear. It's quite fitting that modern rope bondage, which combines sensual restraint with power and raw elegance, has roots in martial arts, which is built on the same fluidity, strength, and prudence. *Hojōjutsu* was, however, also used as a way to immobilize and humiliate prisoners and to demonstrate the captors' power over their captives. It is this blending of art and power play that makes modern rope bondage the exciting and incredibly sexy practice it is today. It is important to remember that the militaristic origins of rope bondage have about as much in common with its sensual development as chickens do with the development of the omelet. We aren't out to hurt our partners, just to restrain and have fun.

The prevalence of rope art in Japanese culture eventually led to it turning up in *kabuki* theater, Japan's favorite elaborate and anarchic dance and drama style, which in turn led to rope bondage as a sexual art coming to prominence in Japan in the late Edo period, around the late 1700s/early 1800s. This practice was referred to as *kinbaku*. Combining the rope work of *kabuki* theater and *hojōjutsu* with a new, sensual dimension, *kinbaku*, meaning "tight binding," first brought the sexual element into the art of rope in Japan.

The popularity of modern Eastern-style rope bondage is often accredited to Seiu Ito, the Japanese painter referred to as the father of *kinbaku*, whose *kinbaku* and *kinbaku*-inspired paintings are as iconic now as they ever were. The popularity of *kinbaku* and Ito soared again in the 1950s, and this cultural passion for *kinbaku* has endured to this day.

◀ *There are many different styles of rope bondage, each with its own unique type of beauty.*

In World War II, there existed something of a cultural exchange between the forces of Japan and Germany, which somewhat incredulously led to the Western style of rope bondage becoming known in Japan. The Western style was more strictly based on aesthetics, and the fusion of this style with the Eastern style was christened *shibari,* with America arguably being the world's largest audience for development of rope bondage today. Cultural cross-pollination happens with movies, theater, music, and dance all the time, and rope bondage is simply another wonderful art form that shares many of the same features of intent and aesthetics and has taken root and flourished with influence coming from both Japan and the Western world. *Shibari* created a dynamic and exciting style that is vibrant and fluidly evolving.

These days, the terms *kinbaku* and *shibari* are often used interchangeably, as it is wrongly assumed that they refer to the same thing. In fact, *shibari* more properly refers to the artistic practice of rope tying for aesthetic purposes, while *kinbaku* remains the correct term for artistic and sexual rope bondage.

WESTERN ROPE BONDAGE

The history of rope bondage in the western world is a lot less prominent than in the east. The first mention of rope bondage in any kind of erotic sense was in the *Nibelungenlied,* a thirteenth-century epic poem most likely from Austria. In the story, Brunhilde, the Warrior Queen of Iceland, is bound and raped by her husband and another, after which she sinks into submission to her husband and never again possesses any of her legendary strength and guile. Okay, I can tell you aren't really listening, and I don't blame you; it's pretty dry in the beginning. But what is important to know is that in the early 1900s, an appreciation for bondage and fetish imagery was finally brought to the Western world by John Willie, an Englishman who founded and published *Bizarre* magazine as a vehicle for his erotic artwork. Around the 1940s, Peruvian painter Alberto

Modern rope bondage is a mix of many styles. ▶

Vargas was also popularizing fetish art with his *Vargas Girls* series, which portrayed sensual, erotic images of women in full-body stockings wielding whips and in other delightfully sinful roles. Vargas is arguably the father of modern pinup, and his works are just as scintillating today as they were back then.

It wasn't until the time of the gorgeous, luscious game changer Bettie Page, however, that BDSM art came to prominence in the west. American photographer Irving Klaw turned Bettie into the first bondage model by having her pose for fetish and BDSM-themed images, which he then sold through mail orders. Incidentally, it appears that Irving's sister, who was his assistant, was the one doing most of the tying up, making this landmark woman the first to be publically tied by another woman. Bettie's dark beauty and the playful-yet-sexual style of these images have made the model an enduring icon for pinup and fetish art over the decades since the '50s, and she still inspires bondage models and rope artists all over the world, as well as famous figures like burlesque dancer Dita von Teese.

The discussion of rope bondage throughout Western history has been much more problematic than its presentation in Eastern history; the marital rape of Brunhilde is certainly not a great platform from which to build a healthy understanding of the role of rope in modern BDSM. This mainstream misunderstanding of rope in BDSM has continued for years. In the 1950s, the French author Anne Desclos, working under a pseudonym, wrote a letter to her lover in the form of an erotic novel. In the novel, the protagonist, O, is brought into the world of BDSM by her dom lover Rene, and it is an exhilarating, thrilling novel in every sense of the word. However, at the end, by achieving full submission, it is implied that O has ceased to be anything but a sexual object, having lost herself entirely, which has caused the book to be hotly debated in the world of BDSM. Isn't this the opposite of what a true submissive seeks to achieve? A submissive seeks to become their true self through submission, not to cease being themselves entirely, so perhaps O should have felt herself truly at one with herself in her role as slave instead of having lost herself within the role. For me, rope bondage is a means by which I become more of the person that I am—and this is exactly why it is so beautiful.

MODERN ROPE BONDAGE

Although there are riggers and rope bunnies who prefer to stick strictly to either the Western or, more typically, the Eastern style of rope bondage, and particularly *shibari*, my own style of rope bondage is an amalgamation of the two styles along with my own tweaks. *Shibari* especially has an incredibly passionate and talented community, and though I love and appreciate the sensuous art of *shibari*, there's just nothing I like more than to take a few bunnies up to my cottage on the weekend and spend a few days figuring out new ways to tie them while they sensually squirm in their bonds. This is the beauty of bondage; there's no way to do it wrong, and there's lots of room for your own innovation. Only safety is the ruling common denominator.

That's not to say, however, that there are no rules in rope bondage. In fact, there are many and just as many conventions. As with any activity in which one person takes responsibility for another's health and well-being, there are certain guidelines that have to be known and adhered to so that the only injuries sustained during a scene are the lashes from a cane or a strained eardrum from listening to your submissive beg for mercy. We'll talk about these in the next chapter.

There are, of course, artistic rules of aesthetics as well. Just as a photographer learns the rule of thirds, riggers must know the basic rules of bondage before they can move beyond them. In the words of Pablo Picasso, "Learn the rules like a pro, so you can break them like an artist."

ROPE BONDAGE AS ARTISTIC EXPRESSION

Not every rigger wants to have his or her bunny suspended in midair so that they can explore every dripping honey hole in sight. It's hard to believe, I know, but it's true. Some riggers (and bunnies, for that matter) love bondage simply for the aesthetic value, and though sensuality plays a huge part in this, for the spectators, it doesn't get much more hardcore than seeing a nip slip every now and again. In Morpheous' Bondage Extravaganza

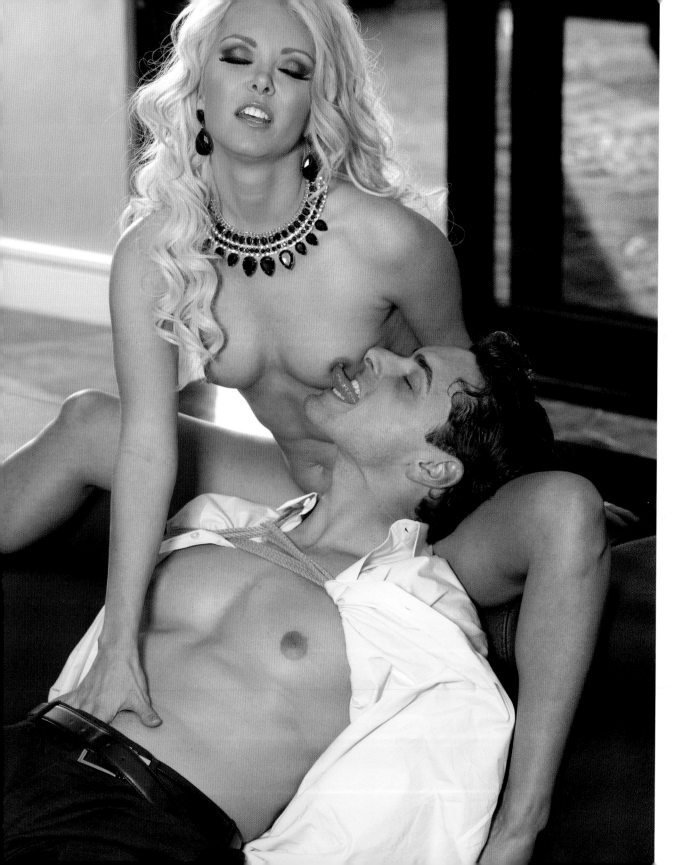

rope bondage performance night, occurring every October, with help from my friends, I make sure that this night focuses specifically on the sensuality and passion of rope bondage alone. For some among us, rope is an interactive art—an art form that has passion, precision, and playfulness seeping out of it at every turn, but art nonetheless. Being a part of this art can differently affect the lucky, luscious souls who are being tied up, of course, but while they're on their intense flights of euphoria, we are confined to just watch.

Every art form, no matter how old, grows and evolves over time—and this is especially true of *shibari*. As mentioned earlier, *shibari* is the type of rope bondage that is purely aesthetic, and *kinbaku* is the proper term for rope bondage that blends artistic rigging with down-and-dirty, filthy sex. Although the untrained eye may not see a huge difference between *shibari* and other styles of rope bondage, there is as much art created in the hands of a *shibari* rigger as there is in the hands of a sculptor. *Shibari* riggers create geometric patterns with their ropes and their bunnies, contrasting the strength and tautness of rope with the soft, pliable nature of the human form—and they make the whole thing damn appealing while they do so.

For *shibari* bunnies, the ties can act as a sort of combination of massage and giant hug—both physical and spiritual. Riggers often ensure that knots are in alignment with pressure points on the body of the bunny, stimulating energy flow and enhancing the chance that the lucky creature on the receiving end of the rope treatment might enter subspace, that illustrious yet enigmatic state that rope-loving bottoms are always excited about. As well as this psychological letting-go for the bunny, *shibari* can also help the rigger to enter an adrenaline-fueled mind space, meaning that the whole experience is tied up in a neat little bow, with the two protagonists engaging in a very sensual experience without any overt sexuality. This will tell in both of their faces, and it can be incredibly erotic to watch, too. I have been tying rope bunnies for a very long time and I still love watching others play and seeing what their creative minds come up with next.

ROPE BONDAGE FOR PLEASURE AND PLAY

The filthier among us (raise your hands . . . I knew it) love the aesthetic properties of rope bondage as much as the next dirty perv, but we also love that a pair of quick hands and some nice red rope can leave our submissives immobilized and ready to be used in any way we can think of. Bondage for sex can be as simple as handcuffs keeping your naughty husband's hands behind his back while you sit on his face, or it can be as complex and intricate as a putting your lithe plaything into a hogtie and suspending her from a specially made rig, just so that you can blindfold, spin, and disorientate her before you tease and appease. Anything that restricts or binds a partner or two (or five) so you can stimulate them erotically is bondage for pleasure.

Although this type of tying is a lot dirtier than *shibari*, it shares a lot of the same beautiful traits, and even when you've a mind for nothing other than the pleasure and pain that you can inflict on your submissive, you'll still be caught off-guard by the pleasing aestheticism of the whole scene. Enjoy this. The beauty is not only in the squirmy lover you have trapped in your rope but also in the fact that they look so damn tasty while you are doing it. Focus is everything; enjoy it while maintaining a foot in reality.

Rope bondage for sexual purposes is even more likely to send at least one of you hurtling into space, as the sensations and intensity are that much greater than with bondage for artistic purposes. For this reason, scenes including bondage for sex—whether that's an elaborate rope tie or simply using gaffer tape to immobilize your partner while she's bent over backward—require much more negotiation beforehand and much more time for aftercare too, for the sake of all involved. Immobilization and any type of restraint that puts the sub in a vulnerable position can bring up a lot of extreme emotions for them, so aftercare should be focused on ensuring that there's a safe, comforting space in which all participants can feel loved and appreciated.

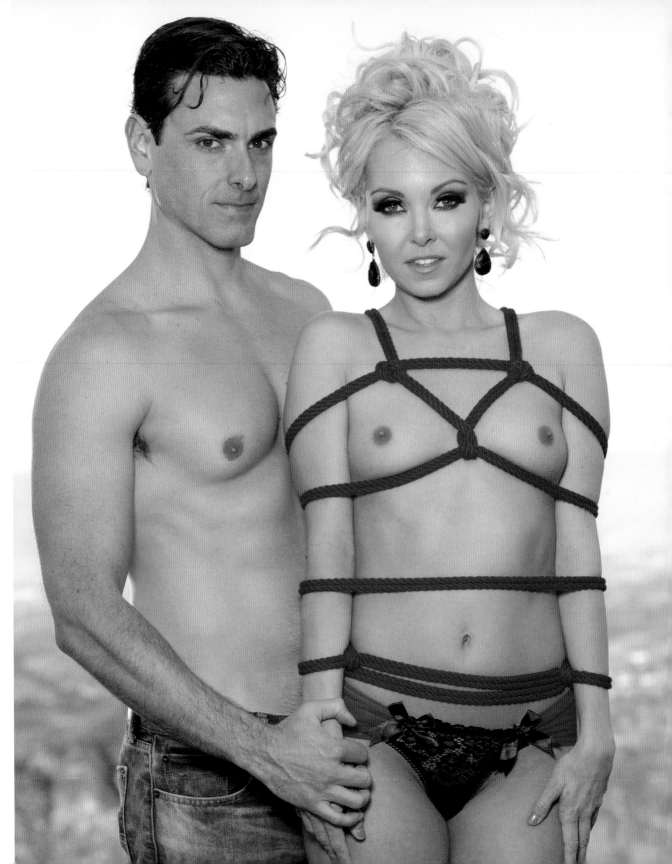

Chapter 3

COMMUNICATION
AND SAFETY

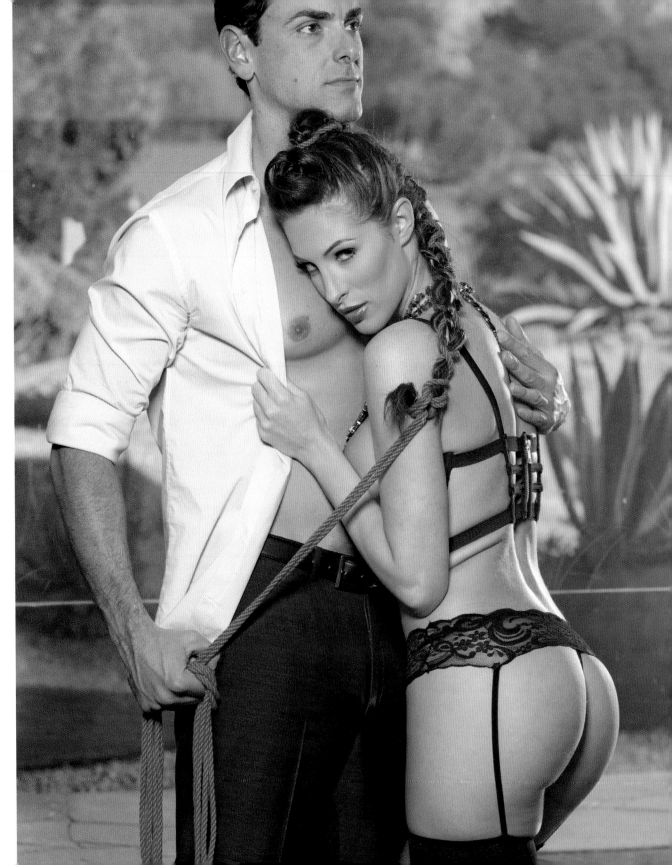

In rope bondage, if all participants don't know the rules, then injuries sustained can be mental as well as physical. This goes for all types of kink and BDSM, and in fact any play, sexual or otherwise, when there's an exchange of power and one party is given total responsibility for the pleasure and well-being of another.

COMMUNICATION, COMMUNICATION, COMMUNICATION

It's something of a cliché, but it's true: Communication is the key to safe, sexy, and fulfilling play. Safe sex is sexy sex. It begins long before the rope is uncoiled and it's still going on when your heartbeats are finally returning to a resting state. In fact, communication should be the constant throughout your whole exploration in rope bondage.

Whether you're taking your first steps into bondage with a partner or partners, going hand-in-hand with someone who's more experienced, or even if you're a single looking to find someone to explore with, your first conversation with any potential partner should be open, honest, and thorough. You should talk about your desires, your turn-ons, and your fantasies, but you also need to talk about your boundaries, your turn-offs, and your concerns. Tell your partner if you're claustrophobic, or if you don't like having your wrists bound together. Tell him or her if you have any medical conditions, like an old shoulder injury from college or a trick knee. Be clear and honest with them especially if you have experienced abuse, mental or physical, in the past. Your partner should also share this information with you, and remember: Though you may not see its significance, your partner will. Always listen and be empathetic. Empathy is key to safe rope bondage sex, and if you feel your partner doesn't value it or has a problem with it, then look for another partner.

Once you've shared your issues, now comes the fun part: Laying down your deepest, darkest fantasies. Talk about those tasty little dreams that will never go away, like your desire to be chained spread-eagle to a thick oak table and used as a sex slave by a group of strangers. Talk about how much you'd love to feel rough rope run down your back,

◄ *Communication is key to any relationship—but it's even more important in rope bondage.*

between your cheeks, and over your genitals before making its way back up to your neck, so every time you struggle, it teases you a little more. Talk about wanting to be gagged with your own underwear while you're bent over and duct taped to a chair, your eyes free to see everything that's happening but your hands unable to move. Share your dirtiest dreams and listen to your partner's. It's the most fun you can have with your clothes on!

When you're finally comfortable with your partner, and you're confident that he or she knows and understands your mind-set, now is the time to start setting boundaries or ground rules. Every person has both hard and soft limits, in life but especially in bondage. Hard limits are lines that you simply will not cross, and that you don't even want to approach in any real way. Your hard limit might be golden showers, or forced lesbianism, or even having your eyes covered; no one will judge your limits, and if they do, then that is not the type of person that you should be playing with at all. Soft limits are a little more open to discussion; they are things that you'll approach in certain circumstances, or things that you'd like to work toward over time with trust. You should know your partner's limits and they should know yours. Write them down, if you think that would help. Some people script out a "contract for play" that sets these boundaries. Come up with whatever makes you feel comfortable that your boundaries will be respected.

Next up is your safe word. The safe word is an essential part of bondage. In fact, it is the single most important topic you'll ever talk about. A safe word is a word that calls all play to a halt. It signals to the dominant participants in a scene that lines have been crossed, and that a submissive is either in pain, uncomfortable, unhappy, or simply distressed. Whatever the reason, once the safe word is said, the scene will stop instantly and the issues will be addressed. For this reason, your safe word should be quick and easy to remember. I like to use the simple traffic light system: green, yellow, and red, with red being the emergency safe word. It is universal and easy to remember. I caution against using complicated words like "flamingo" or "Guatemala" because you might have multiple sets of safe words for multiple partners, and the last thing you need is confusion when all you really need is one easy syllable to get out of the bondage. When one partner is gagged and cannot say his or her safe word, that person should have something heavy to drop onto the floor. This should be something small but weighty. This action should signal to the top that the submissive wants to stop.

Remember your safe word, in case the biting gets to be too much! ▶

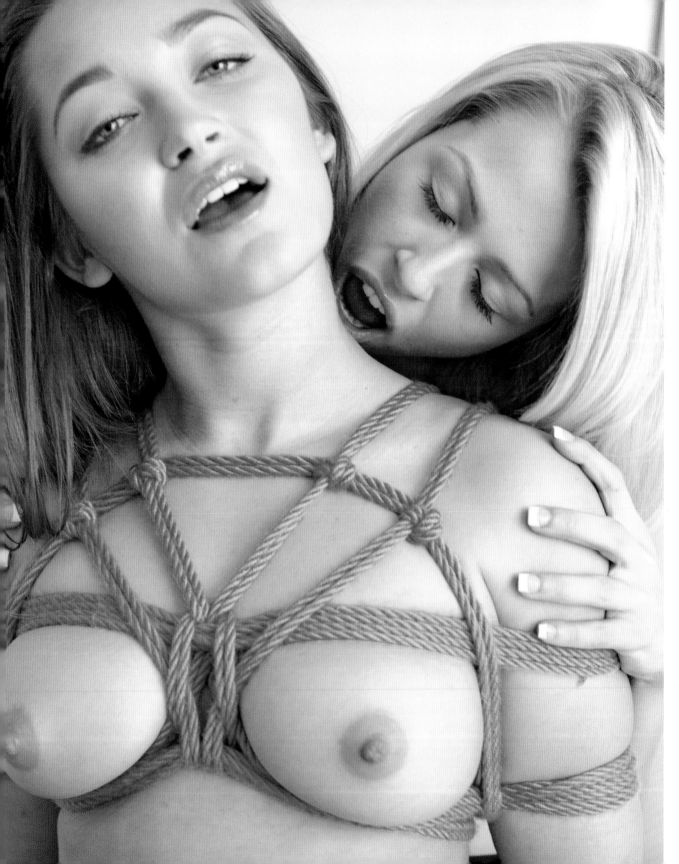

Communication doesn't stop when a scene starts. In fact, good riggers and doms will ensure that communication plays a central role in any bondage scene. You should feel comfortable alerting your top to the fact that the fingers on your left hand have gone tingly, or that your right leg has gone to sleep. The rigger should then handle the situation so that these issues are dealt with, and then the scene can move on. It doesn't necessarily mean the scene needs to end, as sometimes a shift of a rope wrap or a chance to stretch will make everything better and you can continue. If at any time you don't feel that you're being properly listened to, then bring out your safe word. That's what it's there for, after all. Also it is *your* responsibility to be able to use that word when you need to. Your partner is not a mind reader. If you need help, say so. You are ultimately responsible for your safety while your partner is there to support you in being safe.

So let's say that you've been through your first bondage session, and everything went swimmingly. The rope marks on your tender thighs are receding and your dom is feeding you dark chocolate while he rubs your tired neck and tells you how beautiful you are. Lovely—well done you! But you know what's coming next? That's right: more communication. The discussion after a scene is as important as the discussion before it, and as you'll only truly know how you feel about things once they've happened, your journey into bondage will be hindered if you don't reflect on your experiences honestly. Don't be afraid to say if you didn't particularly enjoy a certain something, or if your needs and desires weren't effectively catered to. Be honest and accepting. This is the key to good communication. It doesn't have to happen right away—enjoy that afterglow! Pick up the conversation when the time is right, but don't wait more than a day. You want the memory to be fresh.

PUSHING BOUNDARIES WITHOUT OVERSTEPPING THEM

We talked about hard and soft limits, and how soft limits can be worked toward or even pushed as part of play. But how do you approach your own limits or someone else's without overstepping what everyone is comfortable with? The truth is that this is difficult, and those who are new to restraint should exercise caution in approaching any limits at all. Play partners should have a history of successful play and should trust each other implicitly before they begin to push the boundaries, and you should never rush into it. Remember: There's always another playdate.

I remember one time when I was doing some bondage play and the rope bunny wanted to try a specific position with her hands in a tight tie. Physically everything was going fine, but as we got into the tie together, she realized that she had an emotional trigger from a playdate that went wrong years ago. She quickly said "yellow," so I untied her and then we had a good hug. After a while, we talked about what happened. The partner she used to have would tie her in that position but then engage in emotionally abusive dialog, and just being back in that position brought a flood of feelings, meaning that she couldn't go forward. I didn't know about this when we started (and most likely, she had forgotten about it entirely) but when she said "yellow," I became the compassionate rope partner I am and hugged her until she could vocalize what was going on. The play that evening stopped and we went for dinner instead. That brought levity to the mood and we made a playdate for later that week. We never tried that position again. An easy fix is possible if you are a compassionate partner. Just because the play session ends, doesn't mean it's the end of all play.

If you're the dominant in a relationship, start by asking your sub why exactly they want to approach the issues that surround their soft limits. Some people want to approach these to work through self-doubt or trauma while others simply want to experience something they've always been too scared to try. Understanding your bunny's motivation will help you ensure that everyone is satisfied after a scene.

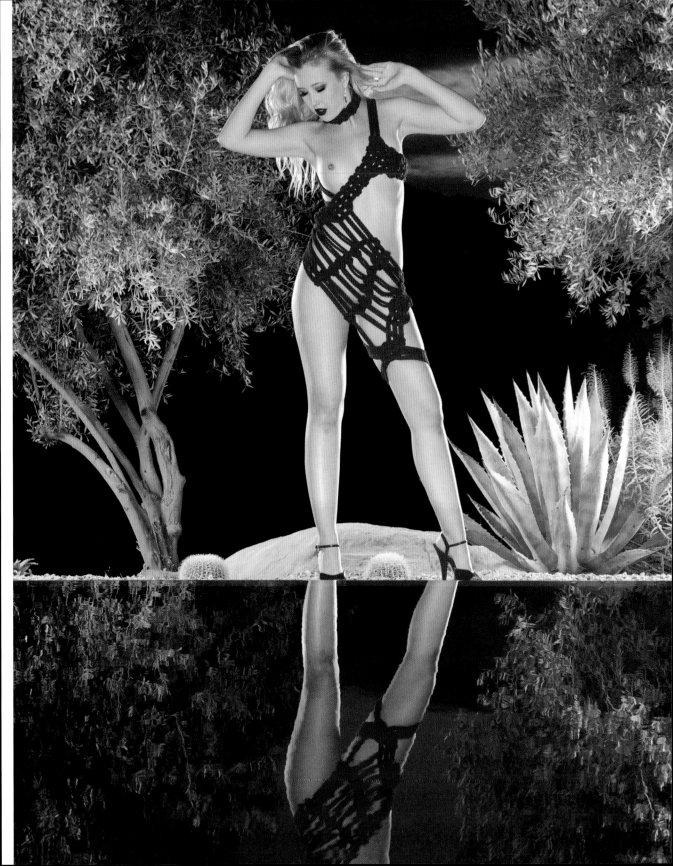

If you're a good top, then it will always look as if you're breezing through playtime with confidence and ease, because you are playing with practiced hands and a partner. But, like athletes, or like a performance at a club or event, there is a lot going on under the surface. As a master, I am constantly on the lookout for any indicators that my sexy, supple subs are uncomfortable or ill at ease, and although I may look as if we have every session planned out to the letter, we will navigate a scene and change tack according to how it's going. Performance is different from what happens in the bedroom or dungeon. You don't have to be Superman, just a super person, when playing. When approaching soft limits, all these skills are heightened and we're attuned to very subtle changes in a sub's behavior. This is part of being a top, and if you're exploring the boundaries of your submissives, you should be attuned to their mood and needs.

I always communicate with my partner during play. It doesn't always have to break a scene; it can be a whisper, a hand signal, or something similar. If you're making a slave beg to be tied and roughed up, you can bring the intensity down for a second to see how calm they become. If he stays agitated, then perhaps you've approached his boundaries enough for one day, and he should be rewarded with something he loves.

THE BASICS OF ROPE SAFETY

All sexual activity has a component of risk, but the very physical nature of rope bondage means that you should play like an incredibly kinky doctor on his day off, and by that I mean that you should always keep safety in the back of your mind while you're acting out your devilish fantasies. Ensure that you know if your partner is fatally allergic to peanuts, or if he has metal pins in his legs, or if she's prone to panic attacks in certain circumstances. You should also think about getting some basic first-aid training if you're a top, as some things can happen out of the blue—and will you really be confident trussing up a delicious new sub like a Christmas ham if you don't know what to do if he suddenly has the first seizure of his life?

◄ *An experienced partner can take you further than you ever imagined.*

Of course, the need for information and basic safety care runs through all BDSM—but rope bondage has its own set of safety precautions. Put in its most simple terms, the central message of bondage safety is this: You should be able to get your submissive out of any restraint in a matter of seconds.

Rope should never cut into the skin too aggressively, and you should be on the lookout for any indicators of bad circulation and worrying discomfort in your submissives. If in doubt about how tight wrist ties are, ask your sub to grab your hand and maintain the grip; if he struggles, the ties need to be loosened. Ties should be snug but loose enough for you to slip one finger in between the skin and the rope. If you're a top, you should always be checking for CSM (circulation, sensation, and movement) in your sub, and if anything seems amiss, undo the ties immediately. There is a risk of nerve damage through overextension or through compression, where rope presses against a certain area and affects the nerves. This type of damage can take weeks or months to heal, so avoid tying around your submissive's joints or making one area bear too much weight. It should go without saying that you should never, ever tie rope around the front of someone's neck, but let's repeat that again for safety's sake: never, ever tie rope around the front of someone's neck.

Good riggers will learn how to tie knots that can be undone quickly, and anyone who restrains anyone else in a device should have the keys for that same device within grabbing distance, but sometimes, it is going to be essential to cut your rope, cuffs, duct tape, or whatever other material your gorgeously twisted mind has decided to use. If you're playing with rope, tape, leather, string, wool, cord, or anything else that can be cut, keep EMT shears nearby. I always buy the ones with the brightest-color handles I can find so that they are easy to see if I need them. They work well on everything that needs to be cut, not just rope—plastic, veterinarian wrap, rubber, etc. If you're more of a heavy-metal kind of soul and you just love chains, locks, and cuffs, you might want to invest in a bolt cutter. If you are a handcuff type of person, keep one key on your regular keychain with your car keys as an extra precaution. Avoid combination locks; it's too easy to forget the code.

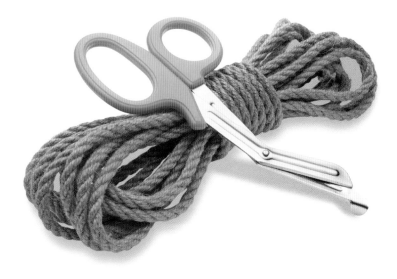

▲ *The most important piece of safety equipment is a pair of safety shears. They are inexpensive and widely available. Don't rely on a knife or a pair of scissors. Safety shears are designed to cut without hurting the skin. They should always be within reach whenever you tie someone up.*

No one likes ruining their toys, and if you've just shelled out for a set of gold-plated leg spreaders for your submissive, you aren't exactly going to be thrilled about setting bolt cutters to them and having some very expensive but useless bits of metal left over (just a suggestion: fancy collars for your cats). If you expect to think twice about ruining a toy or a rope in an emergency situation, don't buy it. Use more disposable ropes or materials. Nothing is more precious than the health of all those involved, and you'd be surprised what mischief you can get up to with ten dollars' worth of wooden pegs and elastic bands from the convenience store on a Friday night.

You should never, ever leave someone alone when they're restrained. EVER. The number one cause of death and serious injury in bondage is someone being alone in restraints. This is nonnegotiable in any circumstance, and if you cannot follow this basic rule of bondage, you should not be playing. It's as simple as that.

Although a glass of good merlot can loosen you up before a scene and help you let go of your inhibitions, it's never a good idea to get out of your head on anything other than endorphins when playing, especially if you're the master or mistress in a session. Impaired thinking is not the friend of safety, so drugs have no place in the bondage dungeon. All partners in all scenes are responsible for the safety of everyone enjoying themselves, so you might be the submissive being used and abused for the enjoyment of others, but if your eyes roll back in your head because you decided to flaunt the rules, you put yourself in danger and threaten the collective safety of the group. Stay sober and don't be a party pooper.

Know the sexual health and history of everyone you play with, and ensure that they know yours. Genital warts are not sexy, and you're going to quickly get a reputation for bad sexual health in the community if you play fast and loose with this rule. Clean and sterilize all toys, sheets, restraints, surfaces, and floors after a session, and be sure to have a bowl of new condoms, dental dams, and water-based and silicone-based lubes within reach for every scene. Stay safe and sanitary for the sake of all involved—and because no one can make herpes look cute.

Play nice, and you'll get to play with all the best people. ▶

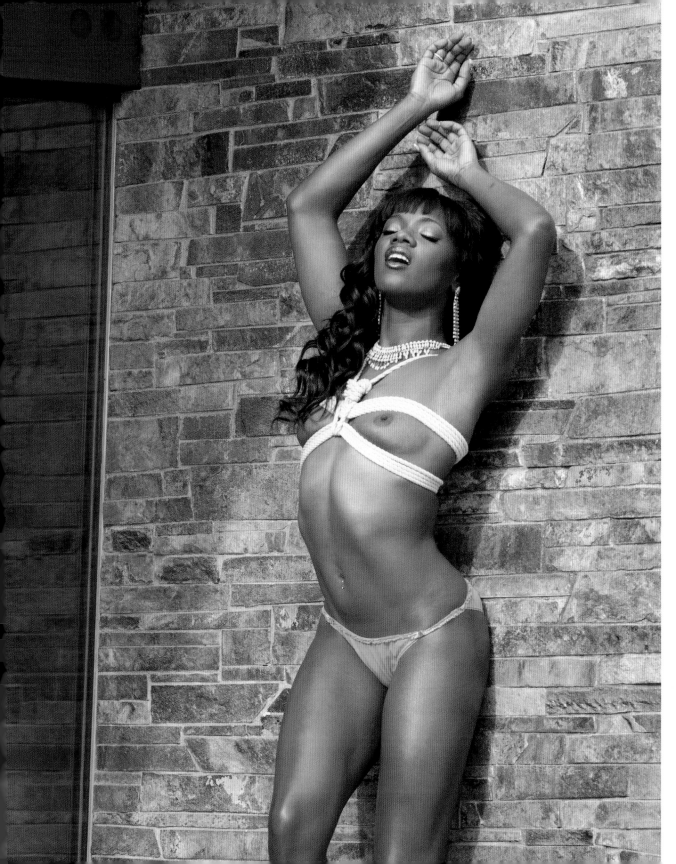

Dos and Don'ts

The biggest two rules in any playtime should be DON'T be an asshole and DO be safe, but in reality, there are a few more things to think about when exploring rope bondage.

DON'T:

- EVER leave someone in bondage alone.
- Let rope cut into the body.
- Make ties too tight.
- Tie rope, cord, or anything else around the throat.
- Buy anything that you won't be comfortable cutting off someone in an emergency.
- Approach hard limits. Ever.
- Drink or take drugs before playtime.
- Play with a partner who you don't trust 100%.
- Ignore someone's discomfort.
- Coerce partners into doing something outside of their comfort zone.

DO:

- Know the health history, sexual and otherwise, of any play partners.
- Warm up before a scene (your muscles AND your dirty mind).
- Always have EMT shears, seatbelt cutters, bolt cutters, and first-aid equipment nearby.
- Check for CSM throughout a bondage scene.
- Engage in good negotiation and communication before, during, and after a session.
- Approach soft limits with caution.
- Be clean and sanitary.
- Practice safe sex.
- Set a safe word.
- Ensure that bondage takes place in a fun, comfortable, and honest environment, in which everyone can let his or her most kinky fantasies fly.
- Have fun playing, but take safety seriously.

REMEMBER: CONSENT IS ALWAYS KEY

Consent is affirmative permission given in sound mind.

Read that twice, write it out, and then read it once more. Say it out loud. Without consent, there can be no play. Consent is not received by bullying and coercing a partner into letting you do something that you know they don't want to do, whether or not they eventually nod to avoid your constant haranguing or whining. Consent is not given by someone who's drunk out of their mind or high as a kite. Consent is not given if you ignore someone's safe word, or if you simply forgot to bring something up in negotiation and go ahead with it anyway. Without consent, it is abuse.

If you are feeling coerced in the middle of play with things that you previously agreed to, you can simply withdraw your consent by saying "red" and "I don't want to continue, please." It is as simple as that, and your partner will respect it.

RACK is the code of conduct in the BDSM/bondage world, and for good reason. The most beautiful feeling in bondage is when you can give yourself over to another person truly and utterly, safe in the knowledge that you will be looked after, ravished, and allowed to give in to all your deepest, darkest desires. For us tops, the best thing about kink is to watch a sub's big eyes look up to you, as the trust shines through even when you're flogging a pair of nice thick buttocks or immobilizing someone's delicious flesh underneath your harsh tape. None of this can be achieved unless consent is front and center of a scene.

They say that with great power comes great responsibility, and whether your power lies in your role as a dominant or in your ability to give yourself up to someone totally, the responsibility that comes with that is to ensure you're a great conduit for the message that consent is key. Don't play with anyone who doesn't value explicit consent, and step in and stop a scene when you believe that one person is abusing another by stepping over set boundaries. Teach by example, and you'll be rewarded with dozens of writhing, squirming kinksters all lining up to play with you. Who said the good guys never get to have any fun?

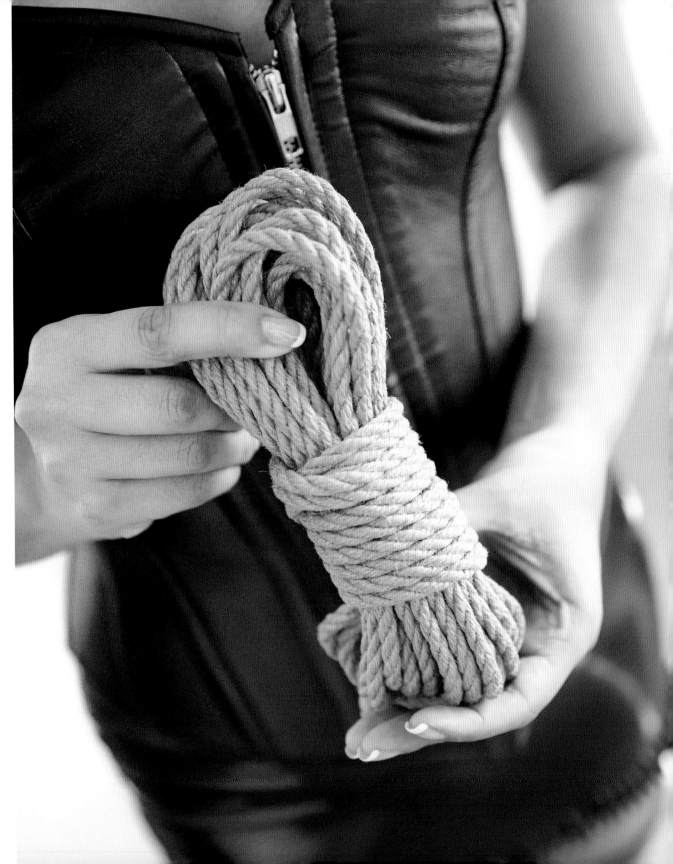

Chapter 4

THE EQUIPMENT— KNOW YOUR ROPE

I don't know about you, but I've always been one of those people who can take a relatively cheap hobby and turn it into something that I spend the vast majority of my income on. My photography equipment takes up half my apartment, and I have more kitchen gadgets than you can shake a stick at.

But when it comes to bondage equipment, even I have to admit that I've gone a little overboard at times. However, it doesn't have to strain your wallet. If your bondage budget only gets you an old rope and two rolls of duct tape, don't worry: You're going to have just as much fun with those two materials as you could with 100 meters of neon rope. Bondage is all about your perverted mind. Toys and materials are just the different tools you have to make those kinky dreams into reality.

In this chapter, we'll be discussing all kinds of rope and other materials that you can use for bondage, but don't be put off by the seemingly endless arsenal of equipment listed; you don't need it all. Just one piece of rope is more than enough to have hours and hours of bondage fun, and you'll be surprised at what you can get for cheap at the convenience store. (Top tip: Get some wooden clothes pegs to nip and tease your slave. You won't regret it.)

DIFFERENT TYPES OF ROPE

There are many different types of rope, but not all are suitable for rope bondage. Though it might seem tempting to just grab that dusty pile of rope that's been sitting in the garage for almost twenty years and start tying your husband up with it, let's first look at the different ropes available and why we use them. (And check that it's not actually a snake that's curled up in your garage. You never know.)

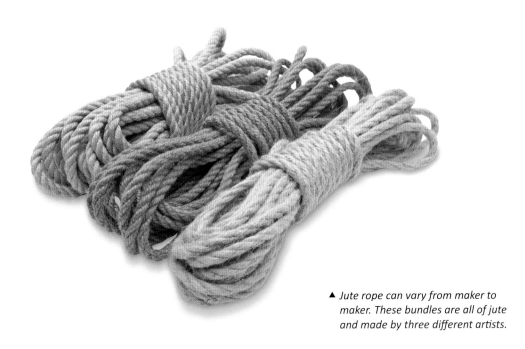

▲ *Jute rope can vary from maker to maker. These bundles are all of jute and made by three different artists.*

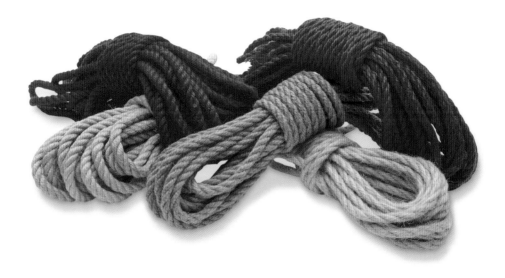

▲ *This is jute rope from four different artists. It comes in different diameters.*

Bondage ropes can be lumped into two basic categories: natural and synthetic. Natural fiber ropes are made of materials like jute, which is a vegetable fiber; hemp, which comes from the same plant as your cheeky little toke at the end of the day (don't worry, we won't tell); and linen, which comes from the flax plant (flaxseeds are also known as linseeds, in case you were wondering where that name came from). These materials are all very hardy, and when turned into ropes, they are twisted rather than braided. They also tend to be pretty rough and abrasive against the skin, especially hemp, so rope makers treat the fibers by boiling and then oiling them, to make them super delicious to use against a lovely sub's skin. Jute is naturally more supple and smooth than hemp, and linen, though gorgeous to touch, is the least often used. The biggest benefit of using any of these types of natural-fiber ropes is that their knot-holding ability exceeds that of synthetic-fiber ropes, with jute in particular being up to just about any task you could think of. For this reason, jute was traditionally used for *shibari*, and practitioners of this type of rope bondage still tend to use this type of rope today.

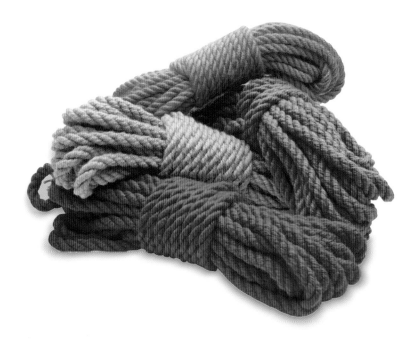

▲ *Cotton rope is a perfect rope to start tying with. It is soft, comes in a great variety of colors, and handles very nicely.*

Of course, the most popular natural fiber for ropes (and really, for anything ever) is cotton. Unlike other types of natural-fiber rope, cotton rope can be braided as well as twisted, which makes it a lot easier on the skin. However, cotton rope isn't as strong as other natural-fiber ropes, and the lack of friction from the material can mean that knots are more likely to slip out than, say, hemp knots. However, the wide availability and affordability of cotton, as well as its softness against skin and general ease of use, not to mention the ease of dying it pretty colors, mean that cotton is a great choice for many nonsuspension ties and binds. Almost all the colored rope in this book is cotton with some bamboo thrown in, so if you like pretty things, you might love cotton rope. You should be able to find cotton rope at home improvement and craft stores, and it won't break the bank even if you get a few lengths of it. It's worth noting here that home improvement stores will become your go-to for kinky sex tools, even though the staff working there won't know why you're dragging home 50 feet of braided cotton rope. Bettie Page was originally tied with braided cotton rope, also known as clothesline, so you are joining a very prestigious lineage.

Synthetic fibers are also very popular for rope bondage, and nylon is the number one material for bondage rope. Nylon is a thermoplastic material that was originally intended as a cheaper alternative for silk, although I'm sure that the manufacturers were thinking of stockings and toothbrushes rather than hog ties and suspensions. As well as being relatively cheap and widely available, nylon rope is smooth, looks supersexy, and will keep its shape when knotted into beautiful ties, unlike some other materials, which will become twisted and distorted as your submissive writhes around. It's also easily wiped clean, and I'm sure I don't need to tell you that that's a positive thing, especially when it comes to ties for sex. More important, it's always easy to untie and won't terrify new bondage partners like untreated hemp will. The only catch is you have to pick it up before you buy it. The softer it feels, the better it will be against your rope bunny's skin.

Parachute cord and thick yarn (shown in the bathtub tie on page 132) are other synthetics that can be used for bondage, but both are thin and relatively weak. They are generally only suitable for decorative knots or for use on smaller body parts. You can use parachute cord to tie fingers together in a scene, or to bind genitals. The added bonus with these two is that you can cut them off and throw them away when you are both done, because of their relatively cheap cost.

Dedicated riggers and rope bunnies will often have a collection of different ropes made from different materials and, if, like me, you're quite visually driven (and can't walk past a nice piece of rope without taking it home with you), a whole rainbow of different colored ropes too. My personal favorites are cotton, jute, hemp, and then nylon. Nylon is a great go-to, all-purpose rope when you are just getting started because it is strong, cheap compared to others, you can dye it with fabric dye (don't forget to set the dye!), and those gorgeous shades that you can get mean that your playtime will always be beautiful. You can hit up local artists that hand-make rope like I do, or others that process and soften the rope so it is ready for use with people.

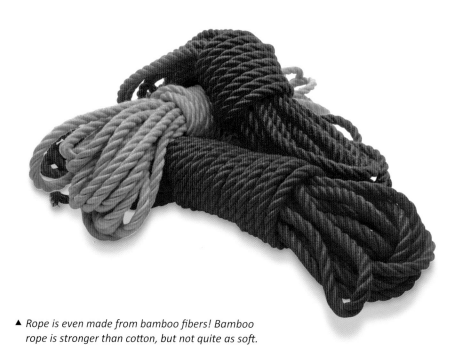

▲ *Rope is even made from bamboo fibers! Bamboo rope is stronger than cotton, but not quite as soft.*

As well as in material, ropes also differ in length and diameter, and unless you want to find yourself halfway through a harness tie with no rope left to finish it, it's important to make note of which lengths are used for which types of ties. In terms of length, anything from 5 feet (1.5 m) to 60 feet (18.3 m) can be used in rope bondage. At the shorter end, you can find length perfect for limb bondage, while at the other end of the spectrum, the longer ropes will allow you to tie beautiful harness ties and suspension rigs. If you're into *shibari*, you'll want to get some lengths cut to around 25 feet (7.6 m) or 30 feet (9.1 m) each, but once you've found your way through the basic bondage ties, there's really no wrong length of rope. Your dastardly mind will find something to bind even with 8 inches (20.3 cm) of string. In terms of diameter of rope to use, I prefer between ¼ and ⅜ of an inch (6 mm and 1 cm) and about 30 feet (9.1 m) long. Rope that's thicker than ½ inch (1.3 cm) can be difficult to use and won't allow you to make the beautiful ties that you crave to see on your supple sub.

All through this book, you will see the natural-fiber rope doubled over and used as one line. This is so the rope can go on twice as fast, and if you need to split directions, you can. There are certain conventions we use for rope bondage, with the 30-foot (9.1 m) length being one of the most consistent. But remember: Rope is just a tool. It is the mind that makes it art.

HOW TO HANDLE ROPE

By now, you'll probably be so excited that you'll have run back from the hardware store, slammed the front door, tossed your clothes onto the floor, and started running your gorgeous new rope along your boyfriend's skin with sinful abandon. But wait! There's still a little more to do before you can leap with reckless abandon into your bondage practice.

Your rope, if cut to size right there for you in the store, is probably going to need to be treated a little before you use it. Usually, it's the ends of the rope that need the most attention. It sucks if you drop a good wad of cash on a nice bit of play material only to have it fray within a few hours and be ruined entirely within a week, so be sure to set a little time aside to make sure this doesn't happen to your rope. If you like, it can be a nice, sexy little teaser task for your submissive to be getting on with before playtime, while you sit and manage the proceedings with a glass of aged whisky and a cigar. Or is that just me?

If you've just purchased a nice, new length of natural-fiber rope, you can finish the ends (or have your submissive do it for you) by simply tying a finishing knot in each one or wrapping each with electrical tape. If you purchased nylon rope, my preferred method is to melt the ends, as this is very easy to do and creates a nice seal. There are other ways to turn raw rope into usable bondage rope, but they're for another book!

Becoming a rope bondage aficionado, you'll want to put your rope away nice and neat for the next time you use it. This technique will ensure two things: (1) The rope doesn't snarl on itself when you go to uncoil it, and (2) you can snap it open with just one hand and you will look like a complete pro.

1. Take the free ends of the rope and make the knots even in one hand, then grab down the rope about 16 inches (40.6 cm).

2. Turn your hands end for end and grab the rope as it falls into your other hand.

3. Repeat until you bundle up almost all the rope.

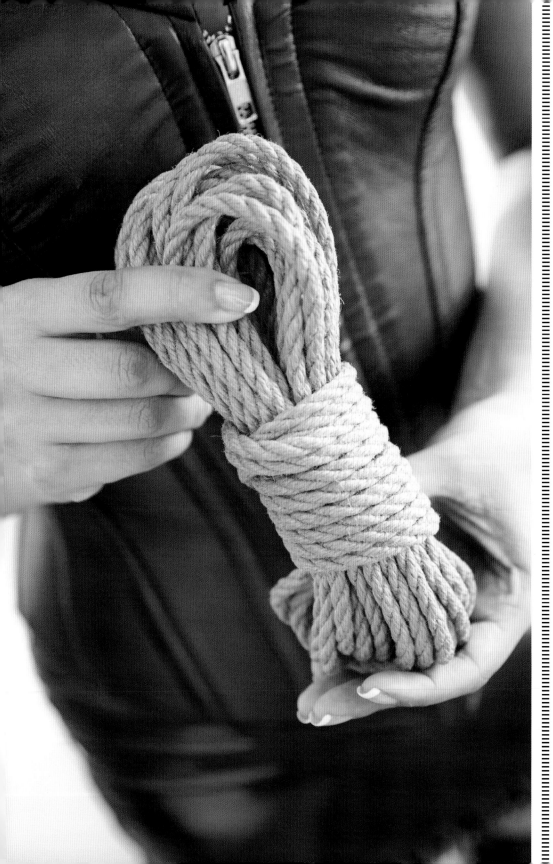
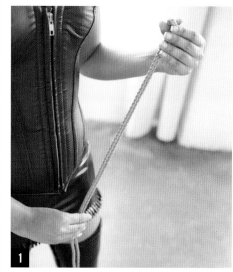
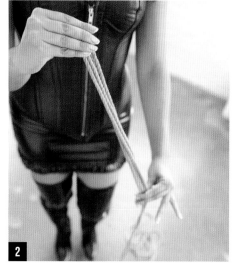
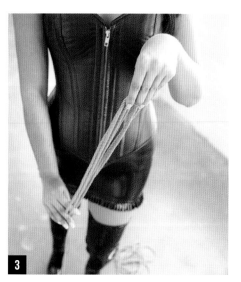

4. When you have about 16 inches (40.6 cm) left over, take the bundled rope and fold it neatly in half.

5. Start at one end and wind the rope neatly around the bundle . . .

6. . . . until you get to about 8 inches (20.3 cm) left over. Then wrap this last section over your finger and come around the whole bundle one last time.

7. Feed the remaining length of rope under the wrap you just did over your finger and tighten the whole bundle.

FINAL: Here you go: Nice, neat, and looking ready for another bondage session!

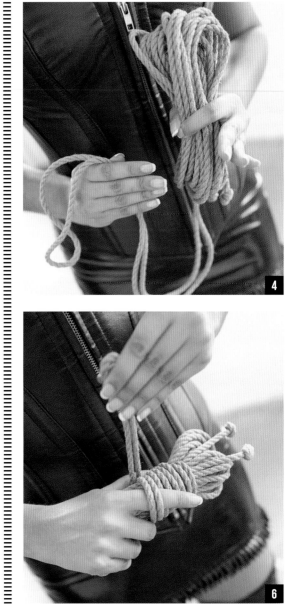
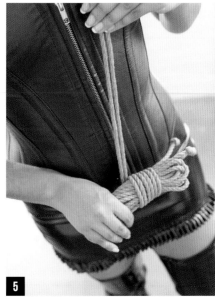
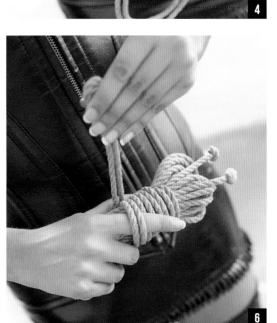
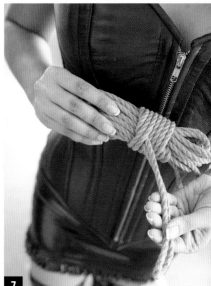

TOOLS FOR YOUR BEDSIDE DRAWER

I'm pretty sure that every adult human has a "toy drawer," and if you're a rope bondage aficionado, then your bedside drawer is going to have a lot more in it than an old vibrator with dead batteries and four different types of lube.

Whether or not you're into rope bondage for sex specifically, the odds are that at some point, you're going to be binding someone on your bed, simply because it's incredibly comfortable and private—and even if you want to rig up your boyfriend just because he looks pretty in pink nylon rope, you don't really want to be doing it out in the family room when Mom drops by unexpectedly. (Worst Sunday visit ever.) For this reason, you should make sure that your toy drawer is always stocked with the correct equipment to keep your bondage time safe and sexy.

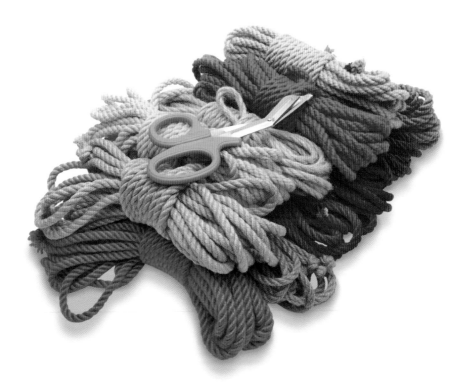

▲ *Rope comes in many different types and colors—as do those essential safety shears.*

As we've already mentioned in the Communication and Safety chapter, whenever you are engaging in even just a light bit of rope bondage, you should have EMT shears within reach at all times, as well as a first aid kit, blankets, and all the other safety equipment we've discussed. Rescue hooks can also be a great investment, as they are easier to use than safety shears and will always get your sub out of a tie immediately. Never play alone.

Anica cream, body cream, condoms, dental dams, and different types of lube should always be nearby during playtime, as well as any vibrators, dildos, anal beads, and any other toys that you might want to experiment with. Remember: Safety is always key!

NONROPE TOYS AND MATERIALS

You can use almost anything to tie a person up in some way. You can use wool to tie a person's fingers, a beach towel to mummify someone, and you can use the ol' classic necktie to bind your secretary's hands to the bedframe while you peek beneath her skirt. Some things are better than others, though, so let's discuss some of my favorite nonrope materials for any scene or playtime.

The least intimidating things you can use to tie someone up with are things that you might usually find in the bedroom, so neckties and long women's scarves are particularly perfect, as are belts and pairs of tights or stockings. Even winter scarves can be used to tie someone's wrists or ankles together, if you're not too worried about killing the supersexy mood with some rough wool or a cozy scarf that your grandma knitted for you a few years ago. One of my favorite bedroom-specific moves involves a pillowcase; turn your submissive over, pull the sub's arms together behind his or her back, make your sub grab his or her elbows, and simply pull the pillowcase up over his or her arms. It's simple, but ridiculously effective!

Scarves can be a nonintimidating and very comfortable way to get tied up! ▶

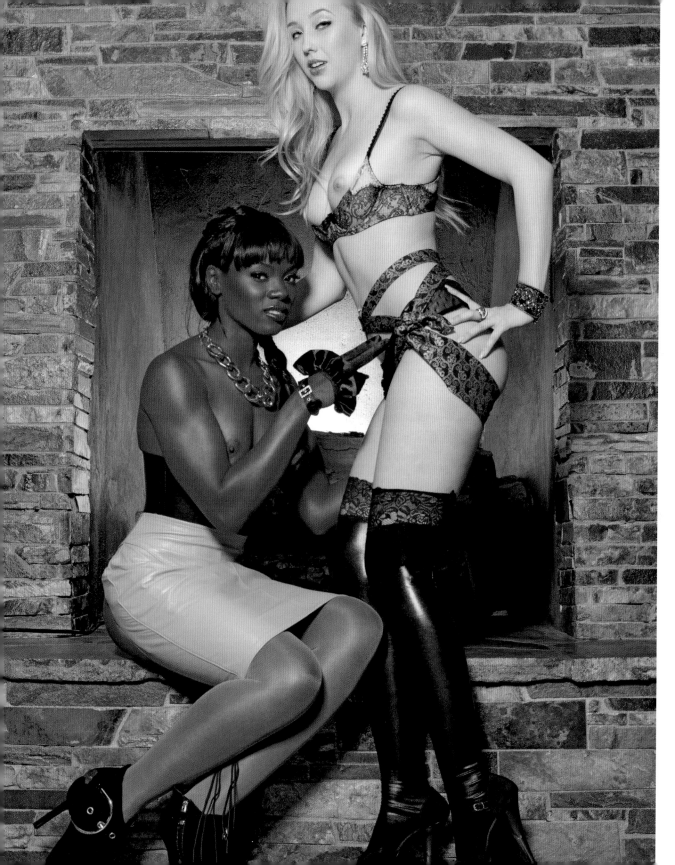

Duct tape is a great little material for bondage as you always have some in the house, but if you love the idea of restriction without tearing your arm (or worse) hair out, then bondage tape might be the perfect solution for you. Bondage tape is especially made for our purposes and doesn't have a side career in hair removal, as it isn't coated with any adhesive; it only sticks to itself. The great thing about bondage tape is that, as well as coming in an array of beautiful colors (mix and match with your rope!), it's reusable as well as wipe-clean. If your budget doesn't quite stretch that far, but your kitchen is stacked to the gills, then you can achieve a similar effect with plastic wrap, but be careful not to wrap anyone's rib cage up too tightly. My favorite way to use plastic wrap is to bind legs so that they're bent back under themselves; this way, your submissive is immobilized but you can still move them around to put them in different positions. Cutting them out when you're finished is also pretty fun.

Of course, there are also a hell of a lot of different premade bondage toys available; in fact, there are probably more than you could ever use in a whole lifetime (although I've given it a damn good go, believe me). Collars and cuffs are particular favorites among the bondage crowd, as these tend to be beautifully made, comfortable, great-looking, and easy to use. For instance, you can splash out on a silk-lined black leather collar for your submissive as a gift for good behavior, and the small clasp on the front will allow you to attach a rope or chain to it and walk her around the house like an impressively housebroken puppy. The same goes for wrist and ankle cuffs. The good thing about these toys is that they're made by perverts, for perverts, so they know exactly what you want to use them for and manufacture them accordingly.

What NOT to Use

You might be feeling pretty confident in your knowledge at this point. You should be! You've learned a hell of a lot in four short chapters, and you should be practically turgid with pride (no, not there . . .). However, although it's important to know what type of rope to use in what situation, it's absolutely imperative to understand when you simply cannot use a rope or other material. This is an issue of safety, and therefore should be at the forefront of your mind in any scene. Using the wrong material in the wrong situation can be incredibly dangerous, so ensure that you understand all the following information just as much as the previous pages.

When you're searching for your first rope purchase, you'll probably come across polypropylene ropes, which are the types used for activities like water-skiing. At first, this might seem suitable, but it is not at all; just touch the rope with your finger and imagine it rubbing against your soft and sensitive parts. It's pretty rough, right? No one wants that sort of chafing when they're trying to get into the zone. Polypropylene ropes are also hard to work with and don't tend to hold knots very well, making them totally unsafe for any sort of suspension ties and otherwise utterly boring. Having your submissive wriggle free because the rope is no good can also kill a scene, so avoid this type of rope entirely.

Climbing rope is another one that you'll probably find pretty early when browsing potential ropes. Make sure you have someone to catch you when you swoon at the price, because this type of rope is about as expensive as it is gorgeous. Climbers, like kinksters, aren't afraid to drop some serious dollars to get high-quality, attractive equipment, but unfortunately there isn't that much more overlap when it comes to equipment. Climbing rope is fantastically strong and durable—as you would expect of something that's meant to stop people from falling to their deaths on treacherous rocks—but it's also too thick to use for bondage and makes knots that are far too big and bulky for our use.

You'll most likely find ropes made of other natural fibers like coir, sisal, and manilla, but these are very rough fibers that don't treat skin nicely at all, and they tend to be incredibly difficult to work with as well. If you enjoy the feeling of a rougher rope against your flesh, I'd always recommend using hemp rope over any of these three; you might like things a little rougher than most, but splintering rope and abrasions on the skin are a recipe for disaster.

Nonrope materials can also be a bit of a minefield. For instance, you might think that an authentic pair of handcuffs, rather than the fluffy pink kind that people always take to bachelorette parties, is a good idea for something to restrain your submissive with. The unfortunate truth is that they are not. Handcuffs are designed specifically to be harsh, uncomfortable, and difficult to get out of, meaning that if your poor partner struggles even a little bit, the metal will cut into the sensitive parts of his wrists and even get caught around his wristbones in odd ways. The worst thing about handcuffs is that you will always, always lose the keys. They're too small, especially when you're both wriggling around getting busy, and you'll end up searching under the bed for an hour while your partner sits there getting bored and desperately needing to pee. There are many other ways to tie your partner's wrists to your bedframe, so leave the handcuffs for the cops.

We discussed duct tape earlier, and this can be one of the easiest and most fun ways to restrain someone on the fly. However, you should never wrap tape around someone's neck or nostrils, and if you bind them too tightly in a nonbreathable material around their torso, they won't have space to breathe properly. Never let yourself get too carried away with duct tape, or indeed electrical tape, gaffer tape, or whatever other tape you have laying around the house. Safety always comes first.

BASIC ROPE BONDAGE KIT

If you're only just starting out in bondage and don't want to invest too much time or money into searching for the right types of rope only to realize that you've got nowhere to hide your purchases, and the cat keeps using your rope as her own personal scratching pile, then, really, your basic bondage equipment might just be a scarf and an old tie (and maybe a pair of long socks, if they're clean). There's absolutely no reason that you can't play around with the concept of restraint using items as simple as this—and maybe some gaffer tape that the builder left.

However, if this type of play turns you on in a way that makes you want to go further, then now's the time to invest in some rope and a few leg spreaders—but remember not to buy anything that you won't feel comfortable cutting through or breaking to release a panicking sub!

Now, everyone's idea of a basic rope bondage kit is different, but here are a few things that I would consider completely necessary for any self-respecting rope bondage lover.

Morph's Beginner's Rope Bondage Bag:

- EMT shears

- 2 pieces of 30-foot (9.1 m) rope, ¼ in (6 mm) diameter

- 1 silk scarf

Morph's Intermediate Rope Bondage Bag:

- EMT shears

- 6 pieces of 30-foot (9.1 m) rope, ¼ in (6 mm) diameter

- 2 carabineers

- 1 men's necktie

Morph's Kinky Devil Serious Rope Bondage Bag:

- EMT shears

- 12 pieces of 30-foot (9.1 m) rope, ¼ in (6 mm) diameter

- 4 pieces of 15-foot (4.6 m) rope, ¼ in (6 mm) diameter

- 2 pieces of 15-foot (4.6 m), $^5/_{32}$ in (4 mm) diameter

- 2 carabineers

- 1 suspension ring

- Scarves and men's ties

- Bondage tape

- 3 leather belts

- A Saturday night with no interruptions

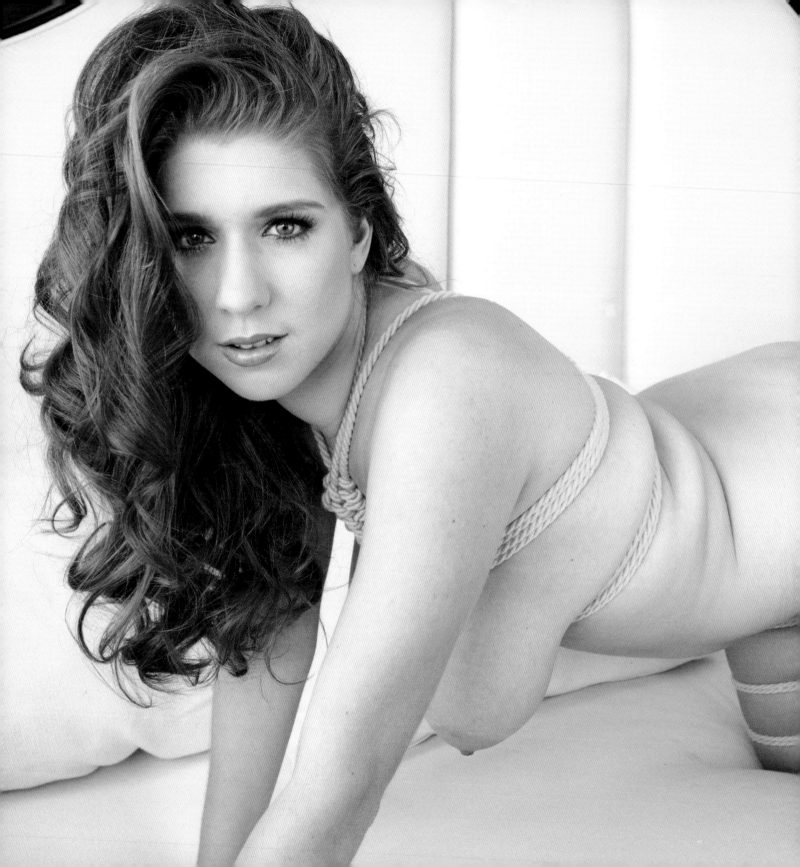

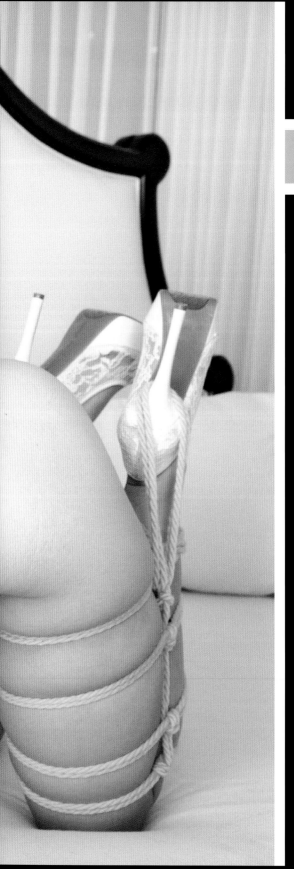

Chapter 5

CHOOSING YOUR BONDAGE PARTNER

Remember in high school when your teacher would announce that it was time for group work and everyone would let out a collective groan? Thankfully, we're all grown adults now, and most of the time, we get to pick who we play with. However, with all the joy of this decision comes responsibility too. No one's going to drop the perfect play partner into your lap, all trussed up and ready to go with a brand-new rope thrown in for good measure. Nope; it's up to you to find a kinky person who loves to be tied up in rope and has all the physical and mental strength that you seek in a rope bunny.

EMOTIONAL STABILITY

What do you look for in a play partner? We're not talking measurements or particular kinks here (although both are pretty enticing), but rather the personality of your ideal rope bunny. As discussed in previous chapters, even for experienced practitioners, bondage can bring up a lot of intense feelings and emotions—for the rigger as well as the person who's bound—and you want to be able to process these feelings with a partner.

If you're an experienced and well-respected rigger, you'll have rope bunnies lining up at your door, in which case it's up to them to prove to you that they'll be fantastic play partners. However, if you're only just getting into bondage, it can be a little more difficult to find someone suitable, especially if you don't know what you should be looking for.

First, think of all the things that you look for in a friend. You'll want someone you like to spend time with. Do you like your friends to have a sense of humor, and do you like to feel comfortable and at ease in their presence? Most likely it follows that these are the traits you should look for in a play partner. Look for someone trustworthy and fun and someone willing to talk about his or her bondage history, sexual and mental health, and what he or she really wants out of your playtime. Look for someone who's open and engaging and without drama. Nobody likes drama.

You should also look for a partner who's emotionally stable and lucid. This isn't to say that you can't play with others who have experienced trauma or difficulty in their lives or those who have emotional sore spots; we have all been through the mill of life and we have the scars and the tears to prove it. However, if your potential rope bunny has obvious issues that he or she refuses to address or seems to be using bondage as a Band-Aid for

No matter what your sexuality, gender, or sexual preferences, there will be many likeminded people in the wider bondage community. ▶

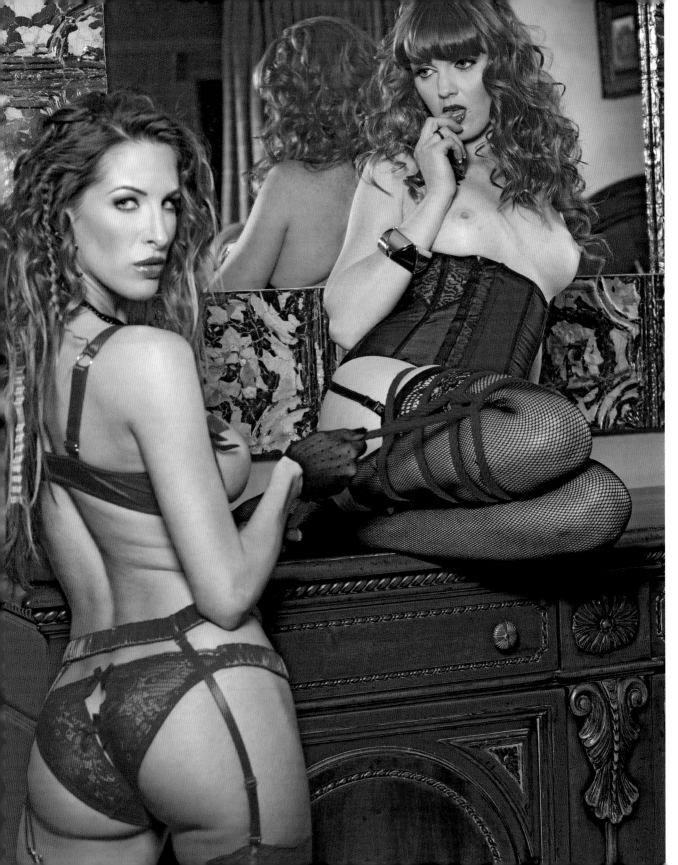

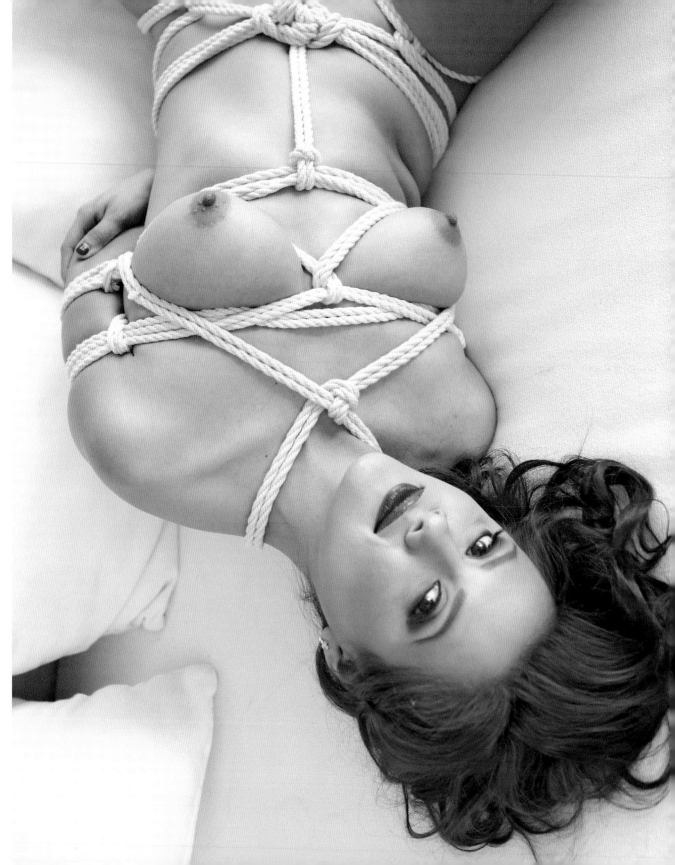

something deeper, politely say no. Rope bondage is often an intense experience, and you should be sure that any potential partner will be able to experience it in a safe and respectful way—and that he or she will have fun!

If you're a rope bunny looking for a top, the same goes—perhaps more so. Be incredibly thorough when meeting with a potential dominant, and don't go a step further than talking until you're absolutely sure that you can trust that person. Outline your hard boundaries, your desires, your experience, and your health, and ask about your partner's. Try to ascertain what type of person he or she is, and if, even for a second, that person makes you feel uncomfortable, politely say no and end the meeting. Ensure that you meet any potential top in a public place the first time, and be sure that a friend knows where you are. Remember that this person will be in total control of your health and well-being, and don't be afraid to be picky. The right top is always worth the wait!

Note: *Rope bunny* is the term used in the community for a person who loves to be hogtied, bound, swung, and displayed, regardless of their gender(s). A rope bunny can be male, female, male-presenting, female-presenting, agendered, or anything in between. Rope bunnies are not necessarily submissives or bottoms; they can be otherwise dominant people who just love to be restrained. We have been using the term *rope bunny* in this book, but if you're uncomfortable with the term, feel free to create your own!

NEWBIES VS. EXPERIENCED PARTNERS

If you're reading this book, I'm going to assume that you're relatively new to the world of rope bondage (or that you're just a big fan—high five!). However, you might be exploring rope bondage with someone who is just as inexperienced as you, or you might have someone in your life who has been in the scene for a long time. This makes a huge impact on how your first steps into bondage will go—and, of course, how quickly you can get down to the really kinky stuff! If your partner is also new to bondage—say, if you're a couple

◄ *Sometimes rolling around on a big couch with a few bundles of rope and your lover can be the best way to spend a Saturday afternoon.*

expanding your boundaries in the bedroom, or if you and a buddy or two have simply decided that your Friday night hangouts really need spicing up—then the key word for you is going to be *slowly*. There's no rush, really; the world of bondage is wide and expansive and there's no need to rush to the finish line (not that it exists anyway, but you know what I mean). If you've never tied anyone up at all, start with something light—a little duct tape around the wrists, maybe, followed by an hour of ravishing, caressing, and teasing, before turning your partner over and taking him or her like you've paid for it. Try all positions and all roles to see which fits you. Build up as slowly as you like, being sure not to push your partner further than he or she wants to be pushed, and when you finally get onto rope, try the easiest, simplest ties first. After your first rope session, allow for an extended aftercare period, as rope can bring out some very severe reactions at first, and don't dive right back into it if your partner needs a little recovery time. There is no rush—and there's absolutely no shame in saying you don't like something.

If you're lucky enough to have an experienced bondage friend, partner, teacher, or top, then your road into bondage will be a little smoother, although not altogether dissimilar. For instance, when I take on a new submissive who is a bondage virgin, if you will, I don't take her straight through to the rig and hogtie her with an ass hook and a ball gag in place. Instead, we sit down and talk. Communication is key, remember, and you should never tie or be tied by someone who you aren't completely comfortable with. We'll sit in a public place over a coffee, a tea, or something a little stronger, and we'll chat about our histories, our experiences, and what we both wish to get from the encounter. Once we're both comfortable and excited to play with each other, we'll plan a date for our first play session. I'll make sure that my new bunny is nice and relaxed (but not stoned/high/drunk), and that my toys don't look too scary or intimidating; no one wants to look a cattle prod in the face on their first time being bound! I'll use a comfortable rope, something soft like cotton or hemp that is less challenging than scratchy jute, and we'll play around a little beforehand, and only when the bunny is mentally and physically ready will we start with some easy, comfy ties. If you're introducing a beginner bunny to bondage, start with the ties in chapter 6. From the first conversation to the final rigging session, we will only ever go as quickly as the bunny wants to. It's a marathon, not a sprint!

HEALTH

Whether you're getting started in rope bondage with a new partner, or starting to tie up the man you've been married to for thirty years, going over the health history of both (or all) interested parties is an absolute necessity before a rope is even uncoiled. For instance, though you might know that your long-term girlfriend broke her leg when she was three and has pins in her calf, she might never have mentioned that she's horribly allergic to grass fibers, and you don't want to find that out while she's suspended in hemp rope and suddenly explodes in a pestilence of hives. Sit down over a coffee and list every health issue you have or have ever had, and ensure that your partner has a copy of this list. This is especially important for those who are playing with new partners. Be sure to include any emotional issues in this list as well. And don't worry—if you have joint problems, heart trouble, or issues with your joints, it doesn't mean that you can't have a very fulfilling exploration into bondage. Even the terminally inflexible with rope allergies can have a tantalizing bondage life. The beauty of bondage is that its range is so wide, anyone can play.

Though you might know your partner inside out (quite literally) once you've tied each other up a few times, remember that it's always important to check how your partner is feeling before a session. Your bunny might have slept funny on his right side, making his shoulder tight, meaning that very restrictive ties around the upper torso might not be a good idea. Similarly, your rigger might have pulled a muscle in the gym yesterday or might have not slept very well, meaning that she isn't as strong as she usually is. In this case, it would be better to avoid suspension ties until the next session.

Once you've got all the information about your partner's physical health, it's time to get down to the nitty-gritty: sexual health. It's never easy to drop a question like, "So, when was your last HIV test?" into a warm, intimate encounter with a potential bondage partner, but it's exactly this question and others like it that you're going to need to ask before anyone gets anywhere near you and your sexuality. Only you can be responsible for your sexual health; don't let others do it for you. You should be upfront about your sexual health, and so should your partner. Don't trust a person who brushes off the question or answers only with "Trust me. I don't have chlamydia." If someone isn't transparent about their past in any way, don't play with them. You should also consider that the nature of sexually transmitted infections is that a person (including you) may not even know that he or she has one, so regular checks should be a part of your social calendar if you're planning to have a diverse and exciting sexual life. And always remember: Play safe!

YOU AND YOUR PARTNER ARE RESPONSIBLE FOR SAFETY

Not to sound like a broken record, but this is worth going over again—and what kind of teacher would I be if I didn't drill the important stuff into your head?

During any bondage session, whether it involves a few simple ties with a silk work tie or an elaborate suspension with three bunnies encased in red rope, every play partner is responsible for safety. First, his or her own, and then the partner's (or partners'). The bondage community is built on honesty, integrity, and trust, and you should consider these traits to be more important than anything else in your journey through rope bondage. Though you might think that, as a bottom, you can get away with slipping a few pills to enhance your experience, you will put the safety of any other bunnies in jeopardy if your body has a bad reaction and the rigger has to turn his attention to you at an inopportune moment. As a rigger, you quite literally have the safety of your partner in your hands at all times, and if you at any point feel that you're not up to the task of dealing with that, end the scene right then and there. There's no shame in getting to the cuddling and caressing portion of the evening a little quicker than you'd imagined—and there's always next time!

No matter how hot and heavy the action gets, safety should be at the forefront of your mind. ▶

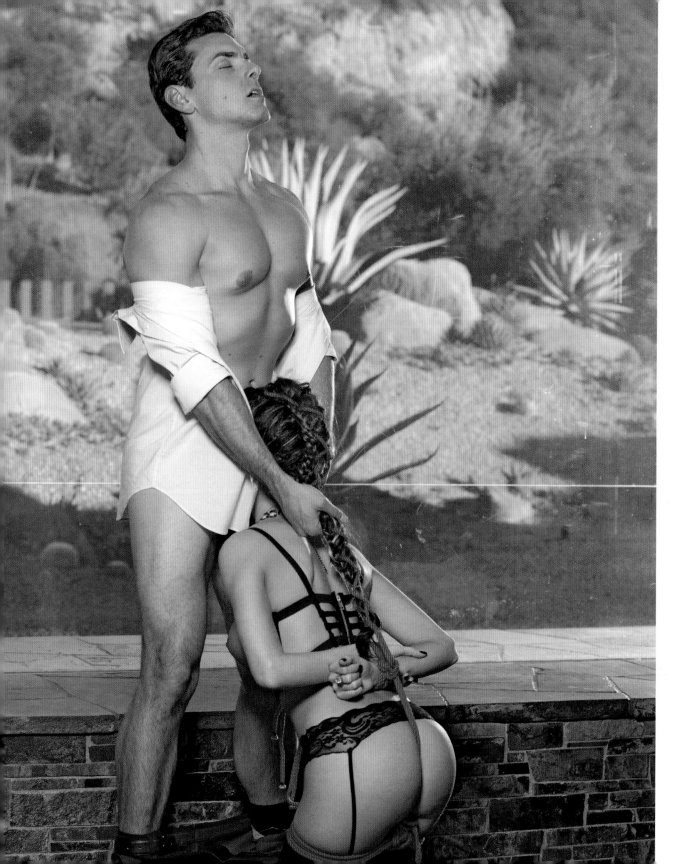

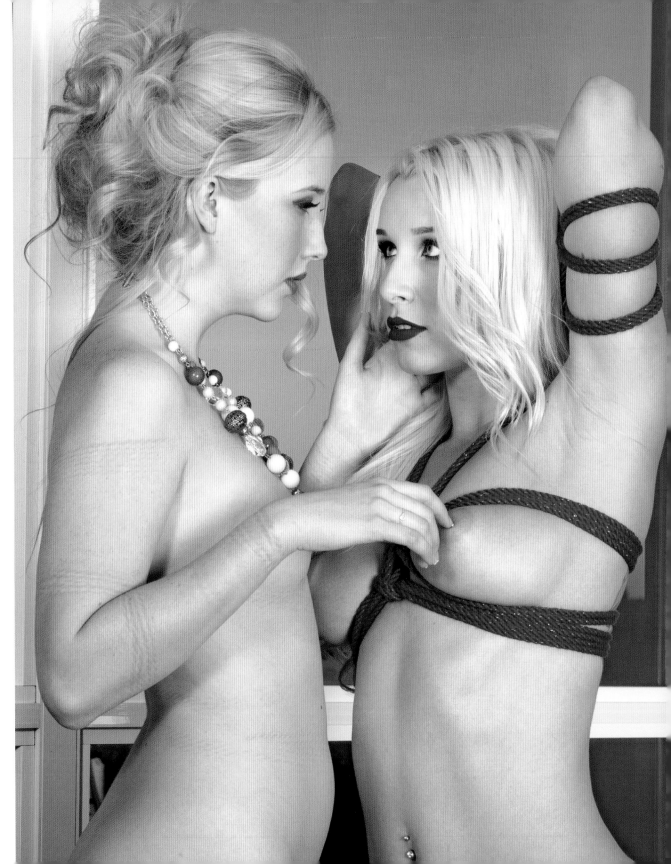

THE POWER PLAY

No, I'm not referring to the situation your favorite hockey team finds itself in when a member of the opposing team has a penalty (please forgive me, I'm Canadian), but rather the exchange of power that goes on when two or more people practice bondage. This exchange is at the crux of all bondage, and of all BDSM, too. This exchange is what makes bondage so fulfilling and fun. For a top, like me, the feeling of having a person give their liberty over to you entirely, even for a brief period, is heavenly; for a bottom, giving their power over to another for a short session allows them to experience great pleasure. For a rope bunny, being bound in rope brings feelings of freedom, euphoria, sexual fulfillment, and joy. For a rigger, being in total control of another brings the same feelings.

All this exciting sexiness can occur because of a thick layer of trust padding any hypothetical sharp edges. Without trust, bondage can be difficult and painful. But how do you know that you're going to be totally comfortable exchanging power with a potential partner?

One great (although somewhat embarrassing) way to figure out how you're going to feel in a power play with someone is to let that person blindfold you and guide you around a public or private place. Let's say that a new top wants to play with you, or that you and your long-term girlfriend are trying to figure out your bondage roles. Go to a fetish- or BDSM-themed event with your potential top, and tell that person that he or she is going to have control over you for a little while. Your top should comfort and caress you to help you ease into the situation, then slip the blindfold over your eyes and tie a piece of string or wool (gently) to your wrist. Let him or her guide you around a little, with that person taking the utmost care to describe what's going on around you and make sure you don't bump into anything. If it's working, you'll feel a little embarrassed but a little turned on; if it's not, you'll feel awkward and kind of anxious. Try it the other way around and see if that's better. If not, maybe that partner just isn't for you. But don't worry; there are plenty more kinky fish in the bondage sea!

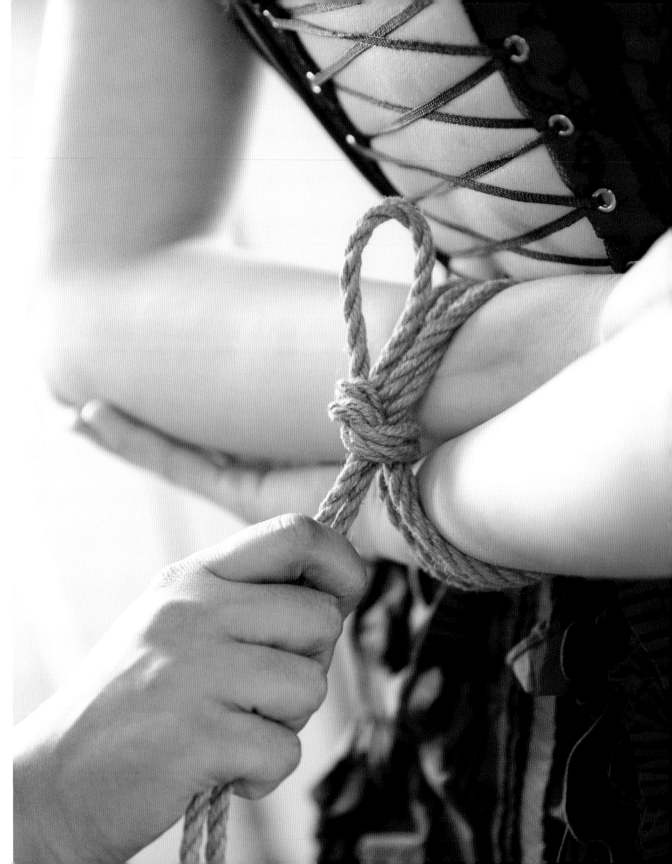

Chapter 6

BASIC KNOTS AND OTHER ROPE PLAY BUILDING BLOCKS

By now, you should practically be frothing at the mouth with anticipation, ready to properly begin your journey into bondage. They say you should always walk before you can run, and nowhere is the concept of progressing in baby steps more apt than in the world of rope bondage. Riggers need to learn basic knots before creating wonderful, sexual, full-body bondage ties. Not only will tying an exquisite body harness make you look like a bit of a newbie if you don't have the basics down, but it can also be dangerous. If you place supporting knots in places they shouldn't go, you can severely injure your sub. Pushing yourself to become better is encouraged—but it's important to also appreciate your own limitations when someone else's safety is literally in your hands.

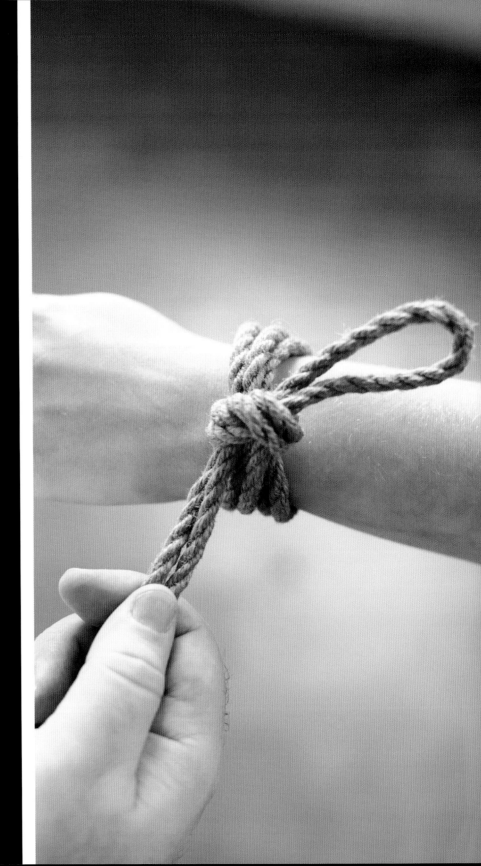

Learn and practice these basic knots: They are your bondage alphabet. Some of you were lucky enough to be Boy Scouts when you were younger. Some were brought up on farms or enjoyed sailing or climbing. Some will have never have touched a rope in their whole lives—and that's okay. For the sake of the total newbies, I'm assuming a prior knowledge of zero—and even if you think you know some of these knots by heart, it won't hurt to refresh your memory.

BULA BULA

This is a classic knot that is the most basic one for starting your ties. It is easy and quick to learn and apply.

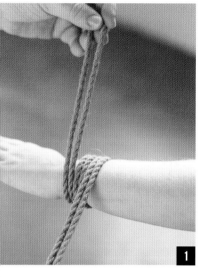
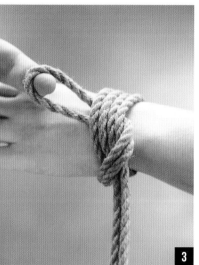
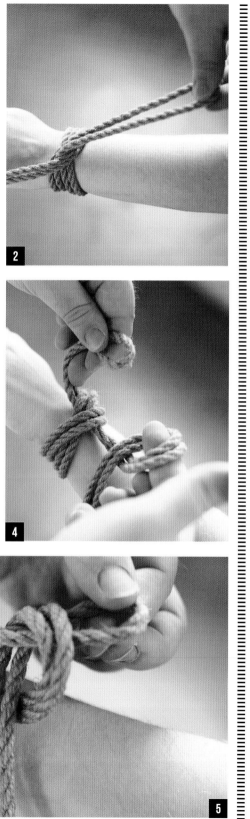
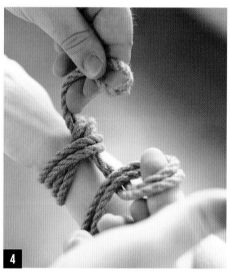
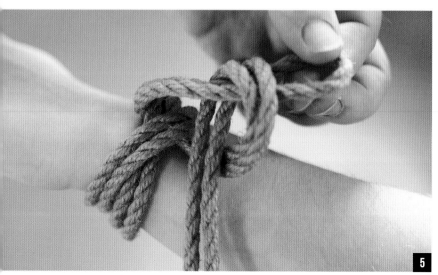

1. Begin by folding your rope in half. Next, take the middle part of your rope and wrap it around the wrist or ankle three times.

2. After completing the wraps, cross both ends perpendicularly.

3. The wraps should be loose enough that you can tuck the short end under the wraps and hook it with your thumb and pull through.

4. Make a loop on the other end exactly in the direction you see here.

5. Pull the short (bight) end through.

FINAL: Tighten the whole knot. This knot has the advantage of being tied quickly and efficiently but is not recommended for rope bondage suspension (that's a whole other book).

LARK'S HEAD KNOT

This knot can tighten down enough that it won't slide along other rope it is tied to. It is what we refer to as a constriction knot because the harder you pull it, the tighter it gets. It is one of the most basic knots and will help you get into artistic rope bondage easily.

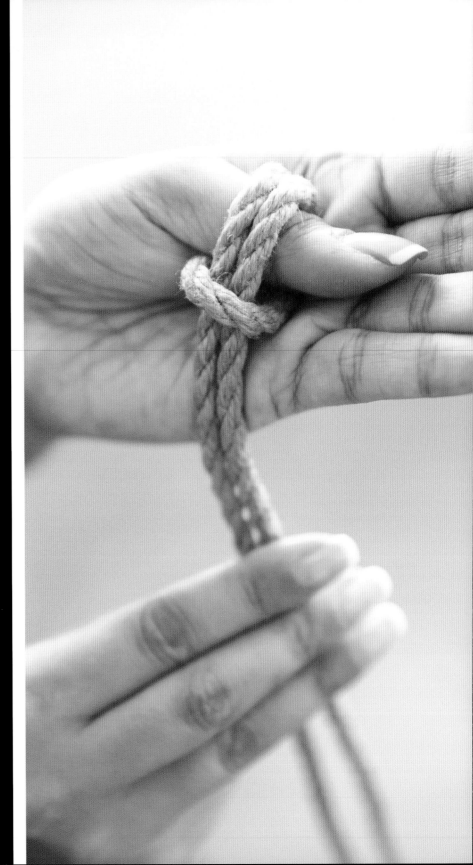

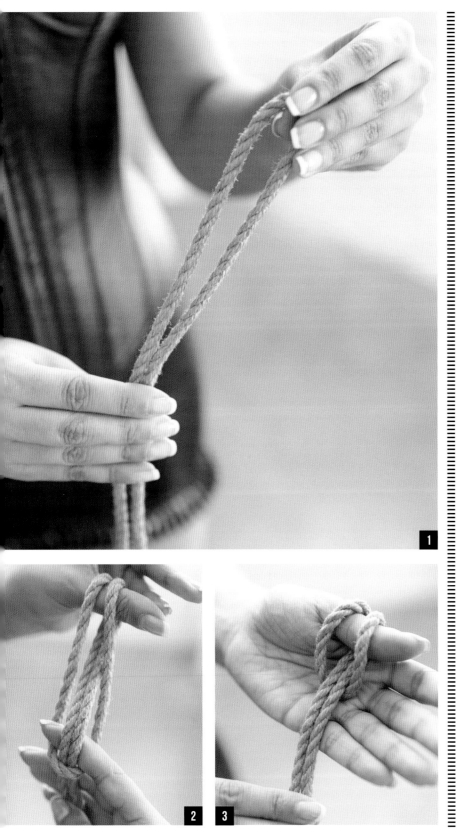

1. Take the middle of the rope in a loop. We call this the bight end.

2. Wrap it around your thumb and pull the long end through.

3. Just like this! This knot can then be slipped over the ends of the rope (coming up in a moment) or be tied in the middle of a rope when you need a tight knot that won't slide around.

FINAL: Here is what the other side of the knot looks like.

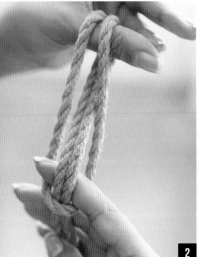

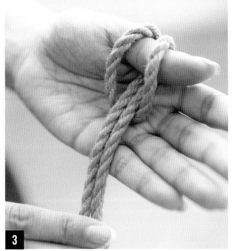

THE MUNTER HITCH

This knot is used mostly for decorative crossovers and changes of direction in rope bondage. You have to keep steady pressure on the knot while tying it or else it falls apart. It makes your rope bondage look more polished when crossing rope than if you just looped around.

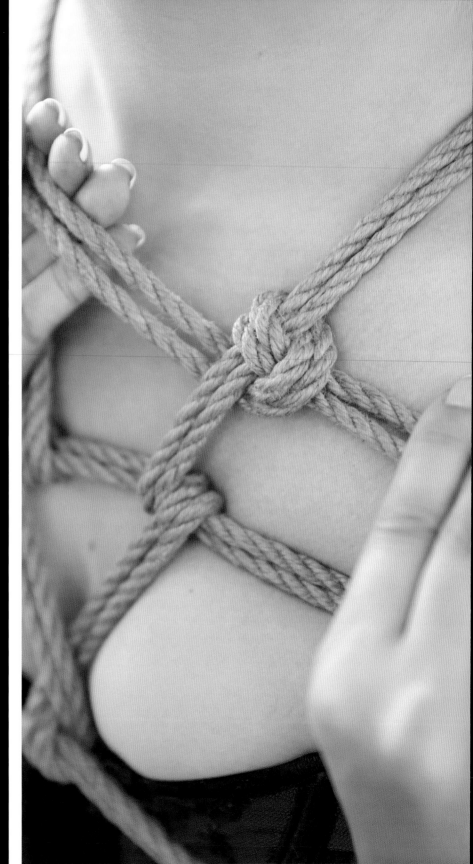

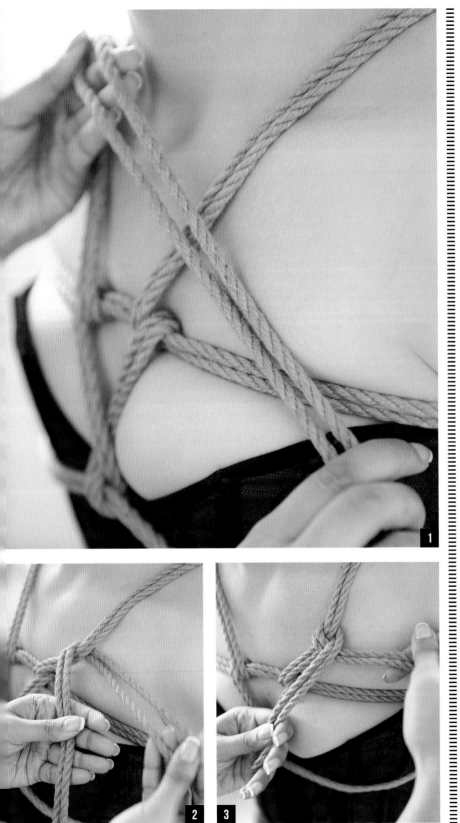

1. Start with the bight end and another piece of rope you want to cross over. Here, our model has a chest harness already tied, and we want to add another piece of rope to carry on a more decorative element. Cross the bight end perpendicularly over the other rope.

2. Bring the loop (bight) end under the rope you are crossing.

3. Now bring it across and over the end of the same piece of rope you are using.

FINAL: Cross back under the rope you just tied around and carry on with the rest of your rope bondage.

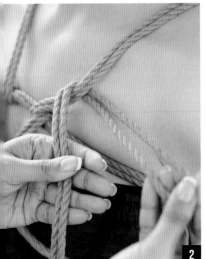

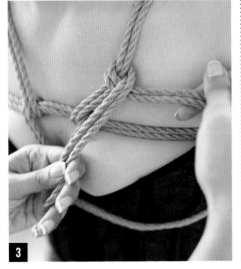

SOMMERVILLE BOWLINE

This knot is a unidirectional knot that is great for starting intermediate ties (generally credited to Topologist in the Western world).

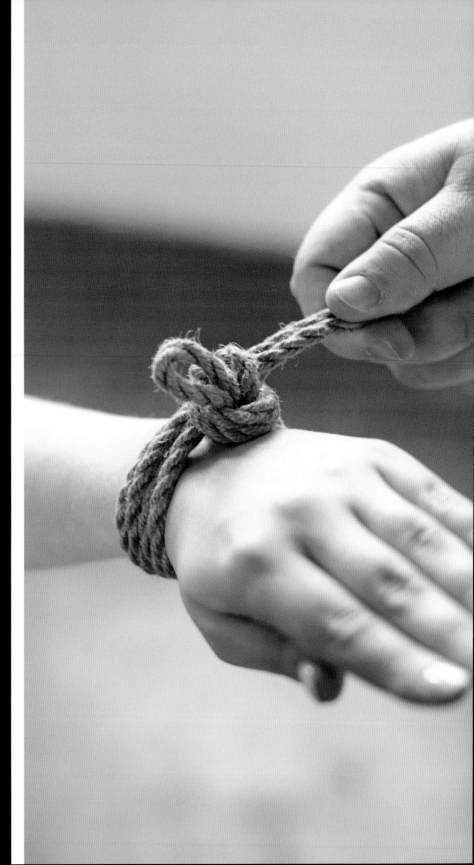

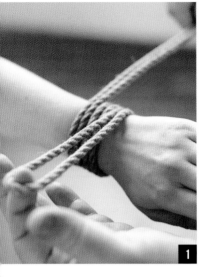

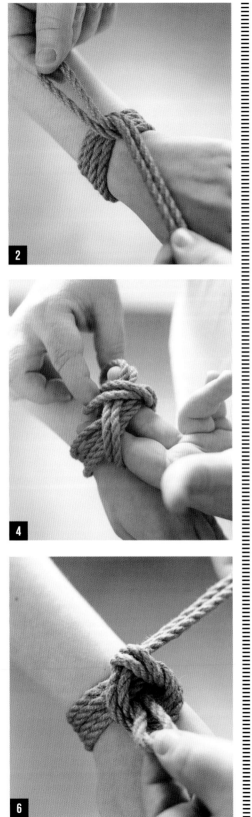

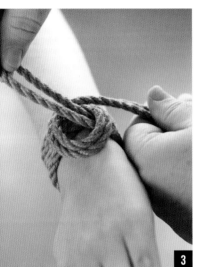

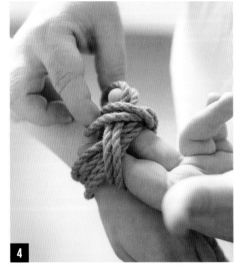

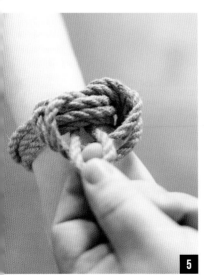

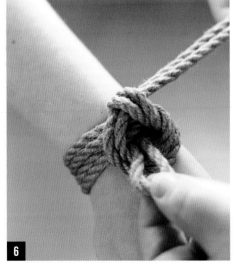

1. Start by grasping your length of rope in the middle, then wrap it around your partner's wrist three times. It doesn't have to be tight—in fact, a little slack is best.

2. Once you have the wraps completed, take the ends and cross them perpendicularly.

3. Holding the short (bight) end, wrap the long end around it in the direction you see here. It is important that the wrap is in the correct direction.

4. Here is the tricky part—but it will pay off if you do it right. Push two fingers through the large loop you just made and under all the wraps around the wrist.

5. Bend the short end backward and grasp it with the fingers that you just pushed through the loop. Now pull that end back through the loop.

6. Now start to tighten the whole knot evenly.

FINAL: Once it is all snug, you should have a rope "cuff" that won't constrict on the wrist. The bonus of this knot is that it holds in all directions and is easy to untie.

JOINING ROPE

Whenever you get to the end
of your rope, you need a nice
tidy way to add more rope.
This works really well.

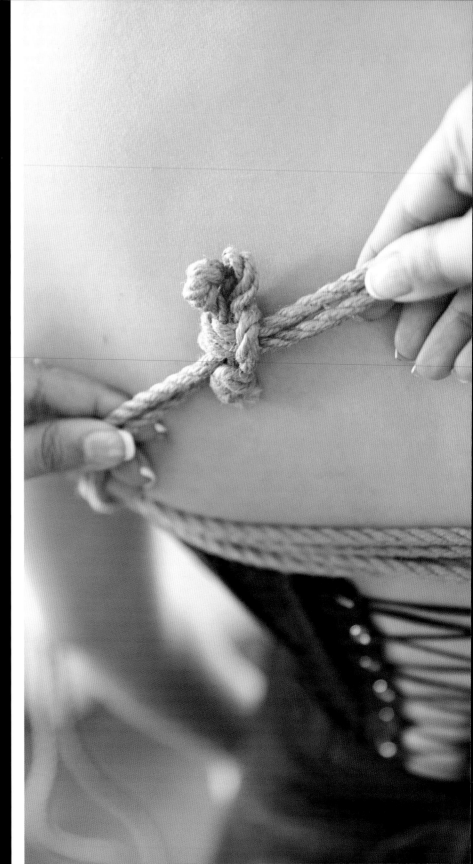

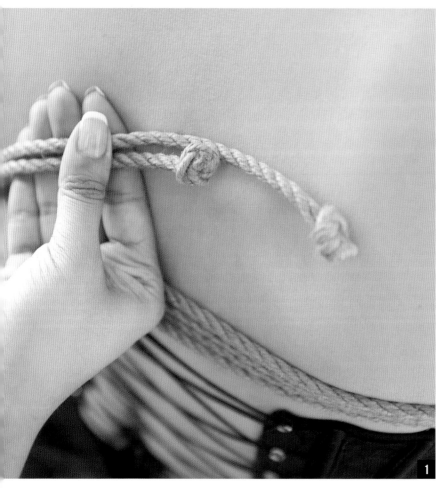

1. The ends of your rope are seldom the same length, even though you started right in the exact middle of the rope earlier. Just like this picture. I don't know why this happens, but I've been scratching my head over it for years.

2. Some people want to just put a Lark's Head around the ends and carry on. This not only makes it look sloppy, but the one end that is too long doesn't have any tension on it, and eventually that slack will be seen in your bondage. There is a very easy fix for this. Take the longer end and fold it back on itself so that the newly created loop end is exactly the same length as the knot end. This is why lots of rope bondage lovers like to have knotted ends on their ropes.

FINAL: Slip a Lark's Head (page 88) around it and tighten it all down. The newly created loop will offer enough bulk to resist the Lark's Head knot from pulling off.

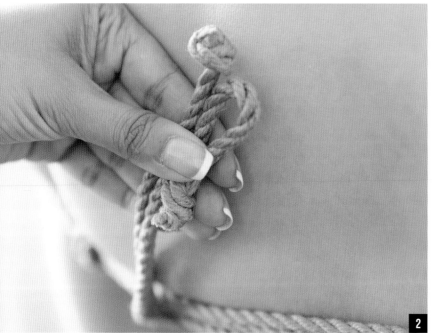

WRISTS BEHIND

This is the only time we tie wrists without any rope in between the wrists. It is because this tie doesn't have to be so tight it cuts off any circulation.

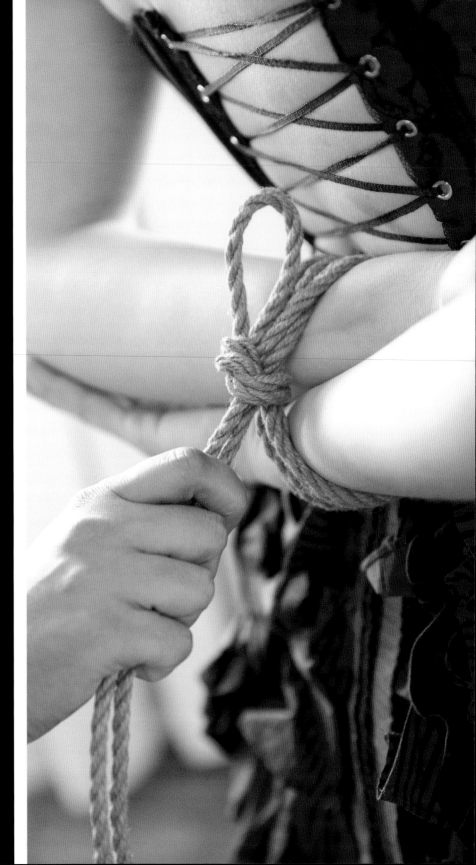

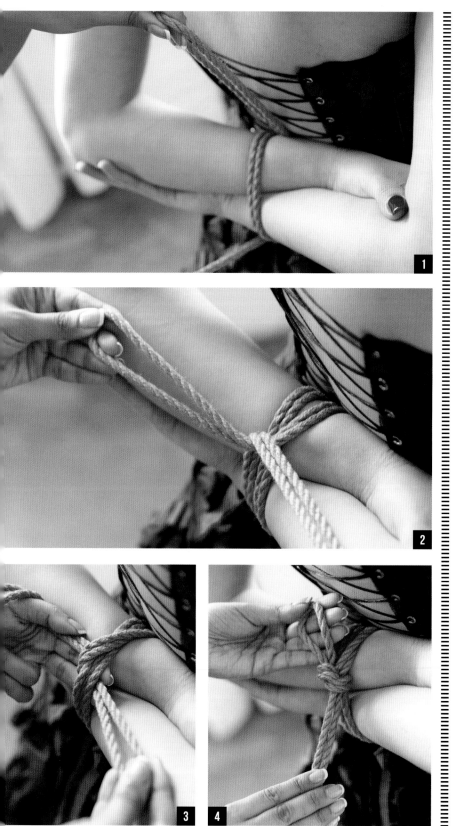

1. Start by having your beautiful partner fold his or her arms behind the back like this. Wrap the bight end around both wrists as shown.

2. Cross the bight end perpendicularly so that the rope has changed direction and is in line with the way the arms are laying.

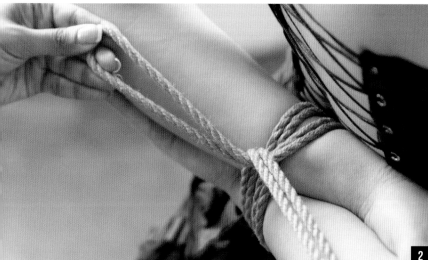

3. You're almost there! Take the loop end and tuck it through the natural opening created by the arms folded together and gently but firmly snug the tie down.

4. Make an overhand knot against this whole bundle.

FINAL: The knot should look exactly like this. When your partner's arms are like this, take care to make sure your partner doesn't fall over. Taking away someone's use of their arms can make them feel off balance. I like to start my ties with this while sitting on the bed.

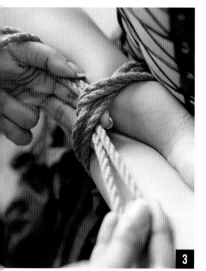

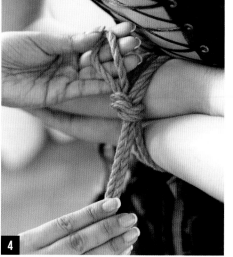

TWO-COLUMN TIE

This can be used for any "two columns" you encounter. Here we are going to use two wrists together.

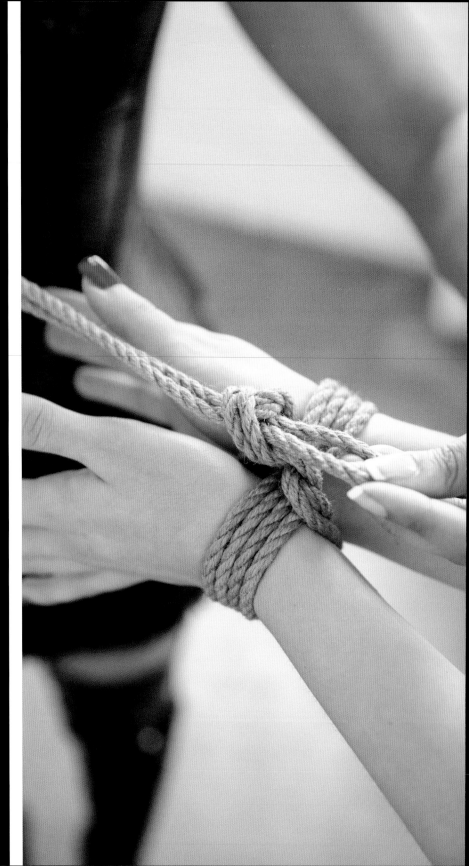

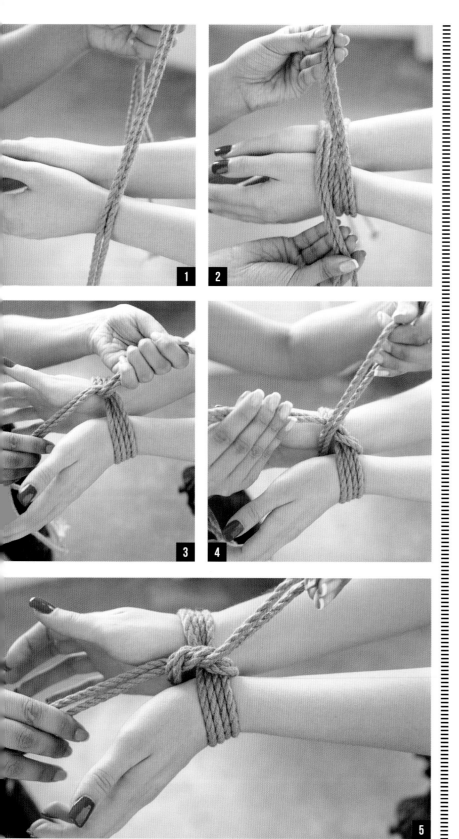

1. Start with the bight end (the loop) and have your lover bring his or her arms together. They don't have to be tight, because there will be rope in between them when we are done.

2. Wrap around the wrists a few times, just like you see here.

3. Now, cross them and change direction (just like the tie behind the back).

4. Now drop the loop end down between the wrists and wrap under and back up so you come up in the center of the arms.

5. Tie an overhand knot. It doesn't have to be fancy.

FINAL: Tie one more knot on top of that.

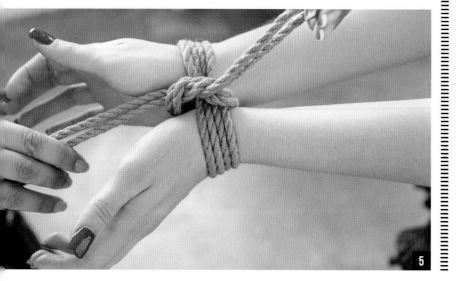

BASIC HAIR TIE

Arms, legs, and torsos are the primary body parts that you think of tying—but one of the overlooked (and most fun) areas of bondage is tying longer hair. This section will guide you through several options for making her (or his!) hair perfectly ready for a nice steady pull, which can be very sensual. With all hair bondage, use a long length of rope or thick yarn. The more loose fibers it has, the better it will grab at the hair. Also, a spritz of hairspray will help the rope or yarn grab better.

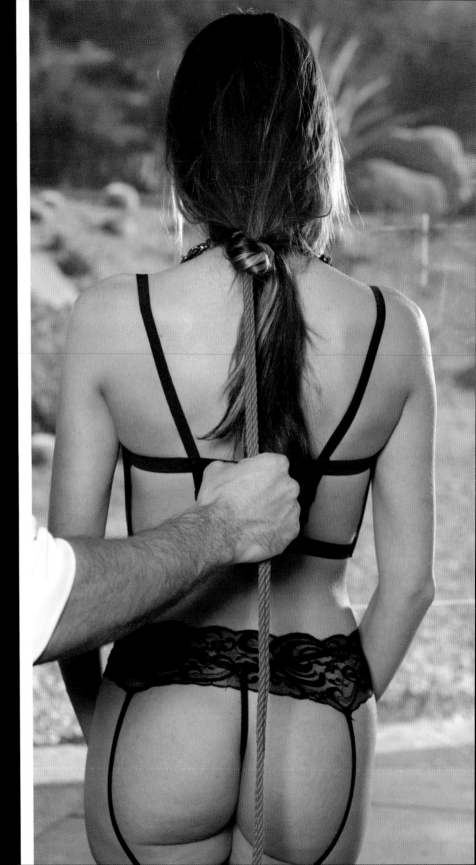

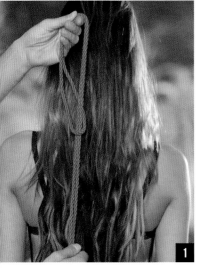
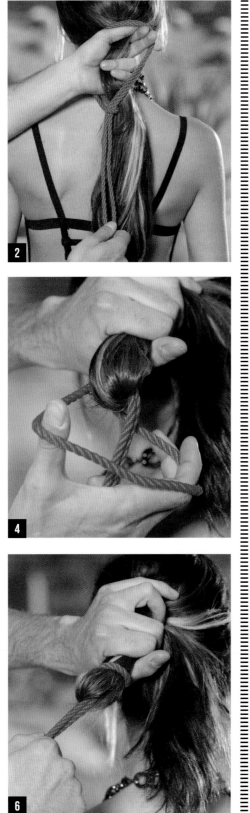
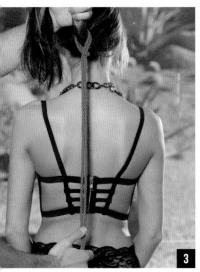
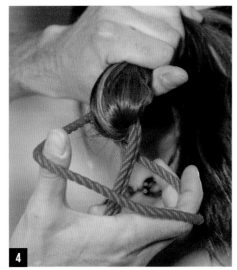
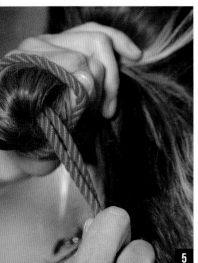
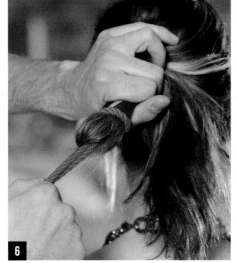

1. A great length of rope or thick yarn to start with is about 16 inches (40 cm) doubled over to 8 inches (20 cm). This is the simplest and most basic hair tie. It holds reasonably well for getting started. Begin with the middle and create a loop.

2. Use a hair elastic to create a ponytail and then grab it firmly but gently. Be confident; she will let you know if you are pulling too hard. Pull the ponytail all the way through the Lark's Head knot (page 88).

3. Push the Lark's Head up over the hair elastic at the base of the ponytail.

4. Fold the ponytail in half and pull the loop open.

5. Push the loop up and over the now-doubled ponytail. If you have done it right, the main line of the rope should be through the newly created middle.

6. Pull it steady! Be careful to not tug any stray hairs.

FINAL: Pull the rope snug and have your way.

TIE

We have seen a different way to tie the wrists together in the foundation ties. This tie is for when you want to cross the wrists. It is very comfortable and easy and very similar to the standard Two-Column Tie seen on page 98.

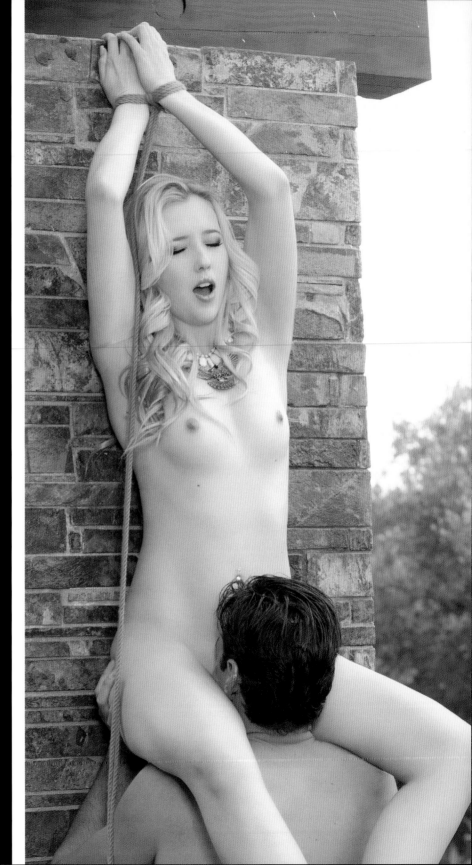

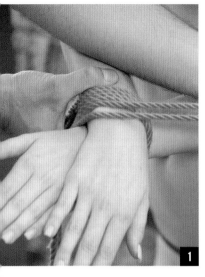

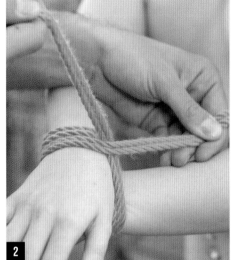

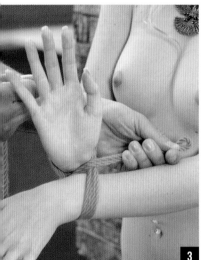

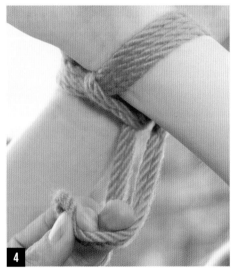

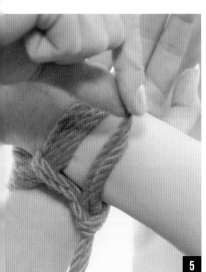

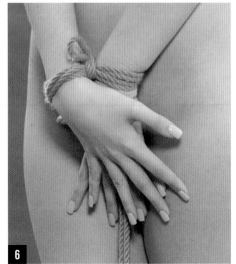

1. Start by making a few wraps around the wrists, keeping the wraps nice and flat, with no twists.

2. Cross the rope right at the base of the thumb. You are going to wrap between the wrists now.

3. See? Just like this.

4. Now come all the way back down and get ready to cross the free end of the rope.

5. Make a nice, easy knot right here.
Tip: Keep the knot in an easy-to-get-at place like the underside of the arms, not in between the wrists.

6. Why don't we add the same tie to the ankles while we are at it?

FINAL: The simplicity of this tie means you can get really creative with positions! Try throwing your partner over your shoulders for a little reward.

NECKTIE SEX HARNESS

Don't have any rope? That's okay! This hip harness uses nothing but neckties to bind your partner into some great ropeless handles for you to grab on to. Everyone has neckties lying around. You can even use long scarves if that is all you have—the knots and pattern are the same.

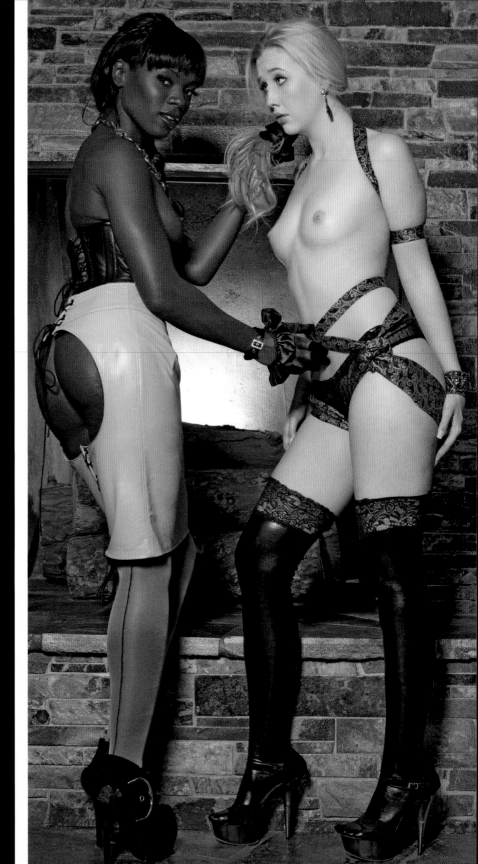

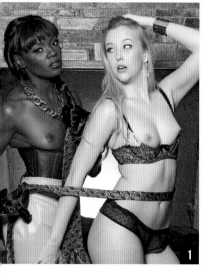

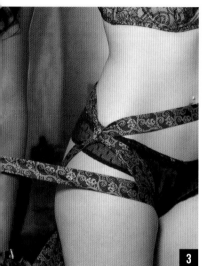

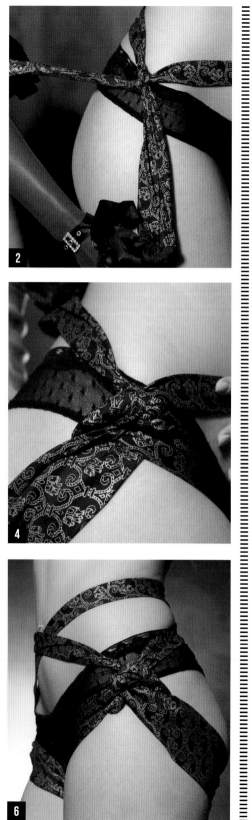

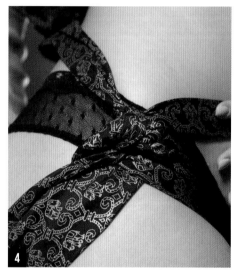

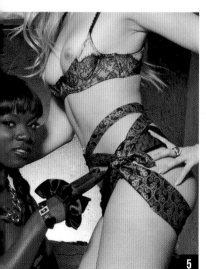

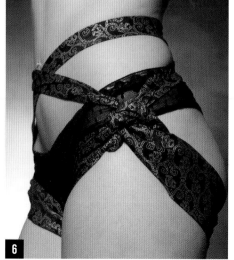

1. Capture your beauty around the waist, right in the middle of the tie.

2. Make a simple knot over one hip.

3. Pay close attention—once you get this, it is easy to repeat on the other side with another tie: Wrap the back end of the tie up between the legs and the front end down between the legs to the back. Make sure the tie lies flat, not twisted. We want your partner to be nice and comfortable in this fuckable hip harness.

4. Come back up and retie a new knot over top of the original one.

5. Repeat with another tie on the other side, making the knots comfortable but not loose.

6. It should look just like this on both sides! Don't forget to tuck in your ends to make it nice and neat.

FINAL: You can complete almost any tie in this book with enough neckties! Make a night of getting creative and experimenting with your lover. Remember to put those ties on her body with authority, and be confident and caring.

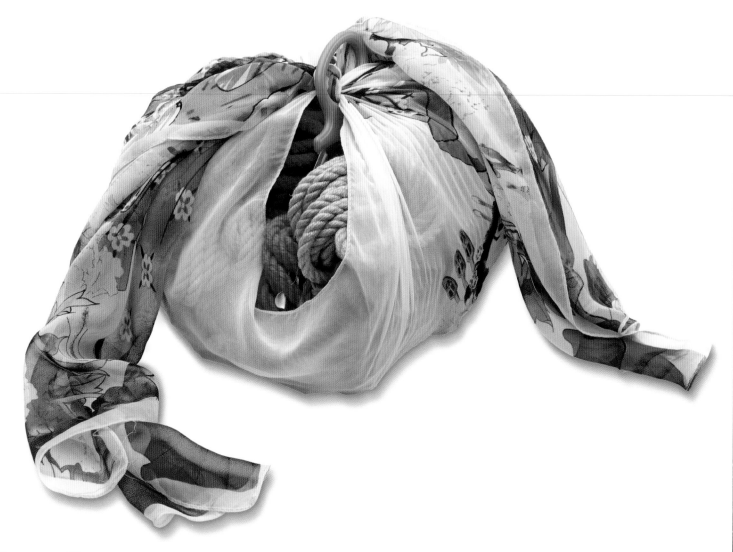

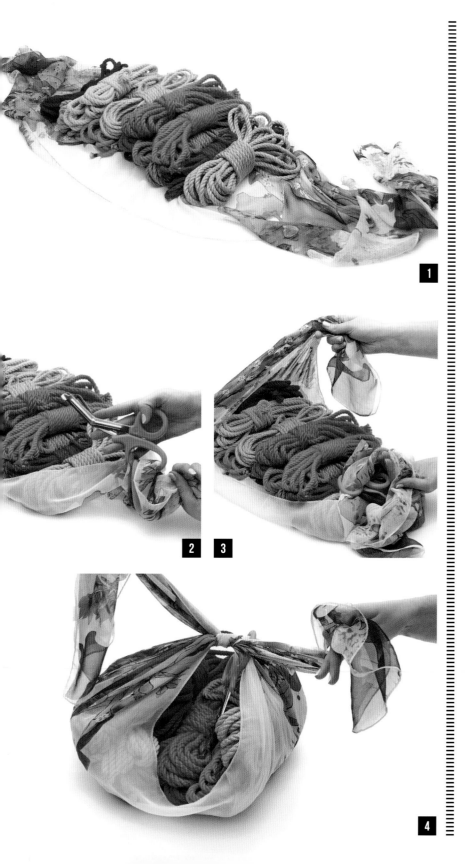

1. Lay out the bundles of your rope on a woman's scarf, leaving enough ends so you can tie it all up.

2. Slide the safety shears you bought for rope bondage (because you are a responsible bondage artist) down one end.

3. Bring the other end over and fold the bundle of rope onto itself.

4. Tie it nice and tight! The tighter it is, the less chance of rope falling out.

FINAL: Nice and neat and ready for the play party—and your safety shears won't get left at home!

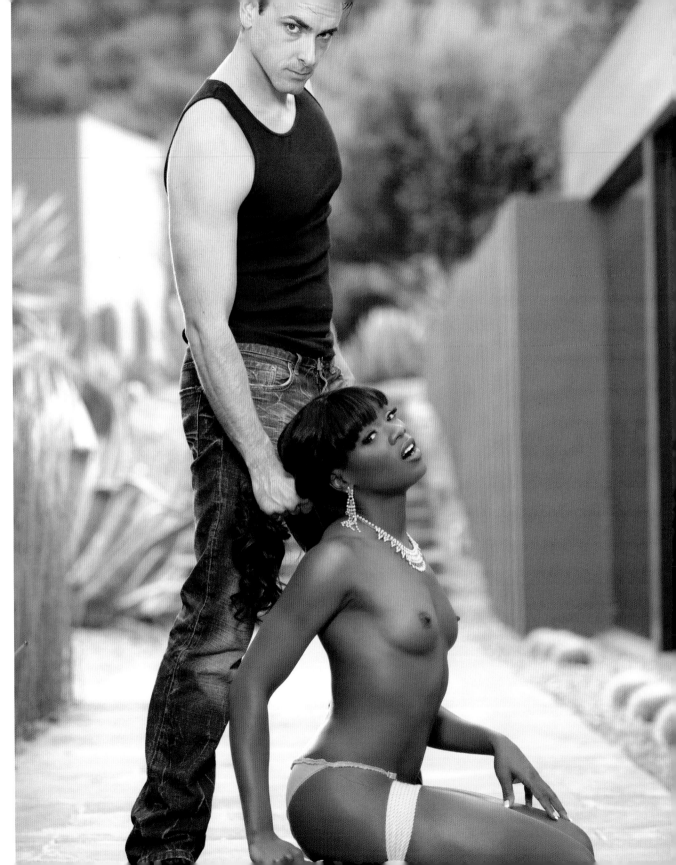

Chapter 7

THE TIES

Now, we get to the good stuff: the ties. Once you've thumbed through the previous pages dozens of times and successfully tantalized your rope bunny on numerous occasions with a simple tie or two, you should be itching to move on to the next level of your rope bondage adventure. If you haven't practiced, then be a good little sub and go back to chapter 6.

We'll start off with some basic ties to use on one body part; this way, you can progress to tying your ravishing partner's wrists to your metal bedframe while you go to town on his nether regions, or tie your slave's arms together, behind her back, so you can play Kinky Police and Rowdy Protestor with her completely at your mercy. You'll see that there are variations of many of the ties—a way to go a little further, or to turn that upper-body tie into a full-body tie. You should practice these separately and together; you never know when your feisty little sub might need a bit of extra restraint! These ties can be used for sex in a number of ways. Of course, the poses suggested here are just the tip of the iceberg; I'll let your filthy mind do the rest of the work.

NOVICE HAIR TIE

This tie is more secure and works well with longer hair, as you will braid the rope all the way through it.

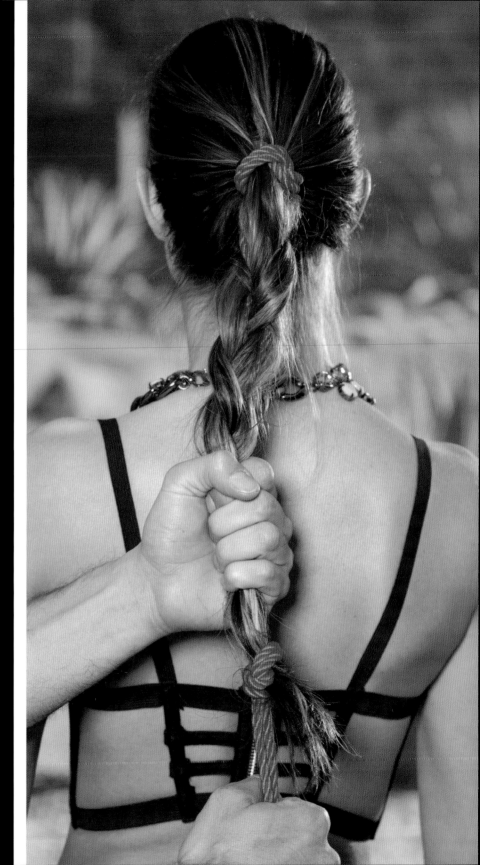

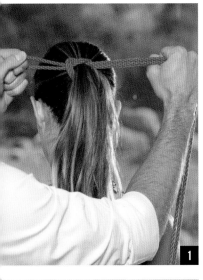

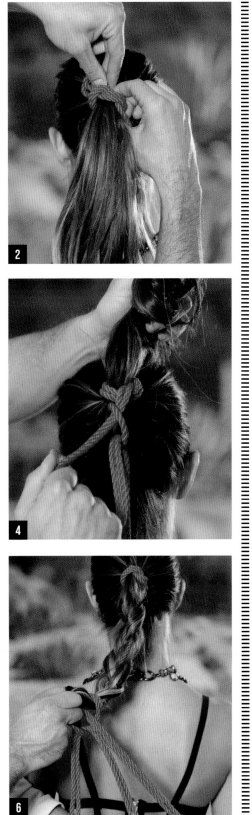

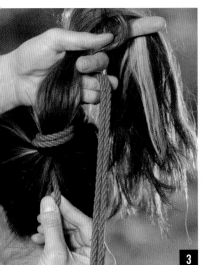

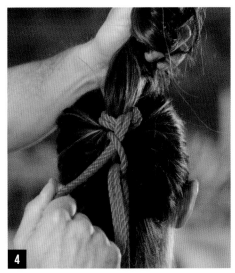

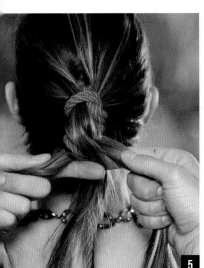

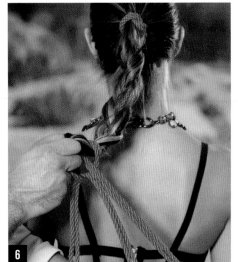

1. Start by taking the middle of the rope and make an overhand knot around the base of the ponytail.

2. Take the loop part and start to tuck it down through the hair above the base of the ponytail, against the head.

3. Lift up the ponytail and pull it all the way through, leaving about an inch and a half down below.

4. Now feed the free end of the rope through the loop and snug it up.

5. You have a firm base to start braiding from. Gather the hair into three sections, put the two pieces of rope into two sections, and start braiding.

6. Braid all the way to the end, then form a large loop and pull it through.

FINAL: Tighten it at the bottom and enjoy.

ADVANCED HAIR TIE

This hair tie looks prettier and will hold about as well as the last one.

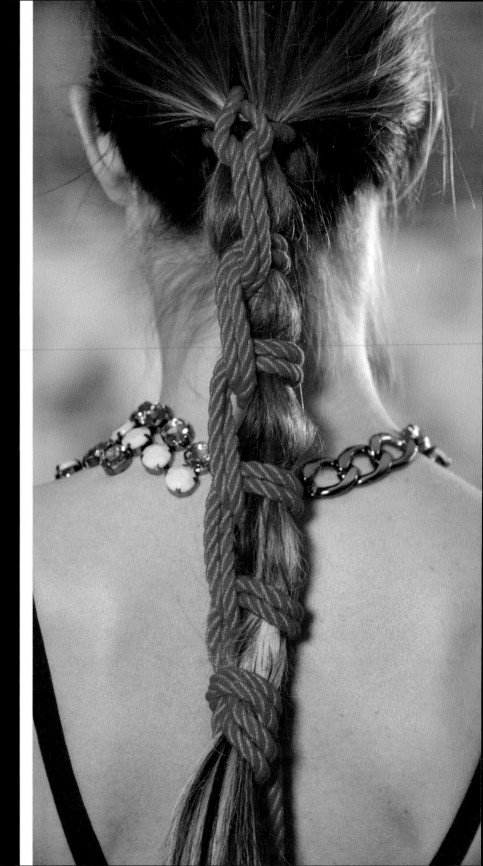

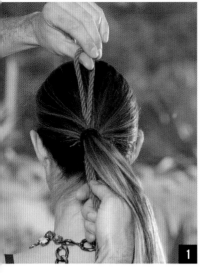

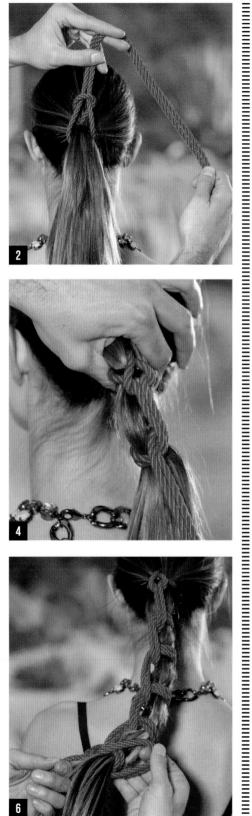

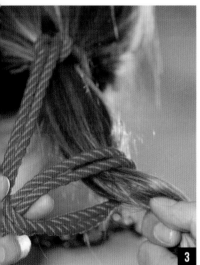

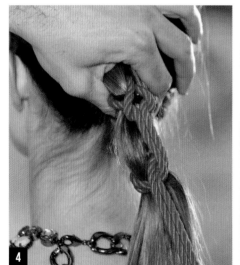

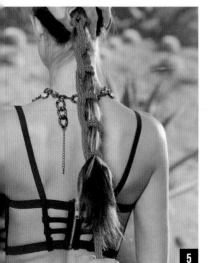

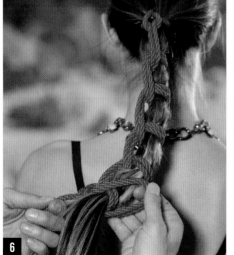

1. Start by pushing the loop up from the bottom, behind the hair elastic.

2. Bring the long end of the rope up over the hair and feed it through loop. This will form a secure base.

3. Now make a loop with the free end on the inside of the loop.

4. Pull it tight. The form of this turn in the rope will hold it in place.

5. Repeat all the way down.

6. When you get to the end, finish it off with an overhand knot up against the last turn in the rope.

FINAL: It looks long and neat, ready for a night out at a fetish party!

KNEELING TWO-COLUMN LEG TIE

There is something very powerful in having your lover kneeling at your feet. This is a perfect tie for getting your partner into a comfortable and proper kneeling position and keeping him or her there. There are many ways to tie someone in a kneeling position, and this is the easiest to start with. It has a nice wide band across the leg, which makes it very comfortable.

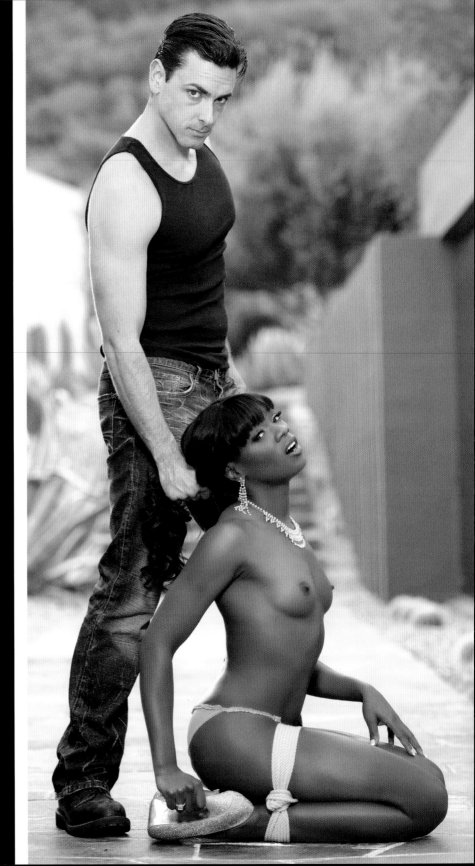

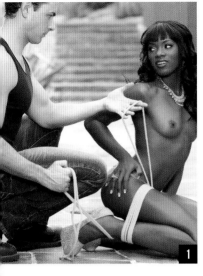

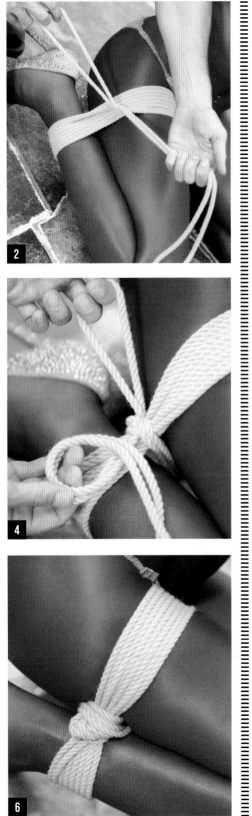

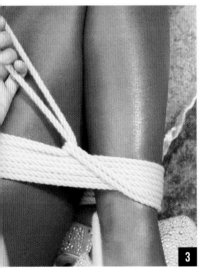

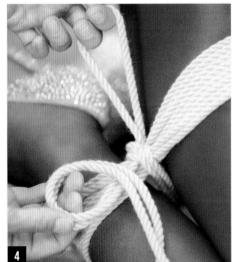

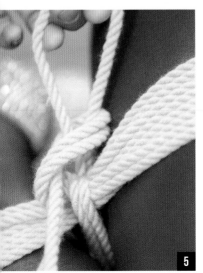

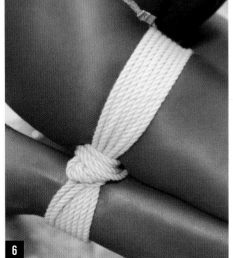

1. Begin with having your partner kneel and make three wraps around his or her leg. You will find it easier to wrap if you keep the wraps up near the thigh because of the space created where the foot meets the leg. It is a natural space as shown here.

2. Finish the wrapping so you have about 14 inches (35.5 cm) left of the loop end. Cross it with the free end.

3. Now take the free end, tuck it down, and wrap it around the other wraps on the other side.

4. Pull it up again and cinch it tight. Now you are set up to finish this as a Bula Bula (page 86).

5. Push the loop over the final free end and cinch it down a second time.

6. Tuck all your ends in. You're almost there!

FINAL: Isn't there something romantic about having your lover kneeling tied at his or her feet while a quiet moan escapes his or her lips?

SIMPLE STRAPPADO

To add a more forceful element, a simple arm binder is very effective at keeping your partner in place.

1. Begin with a basic Two-Column Tie (page 98) around the wrists

2. Bring the rope up vertically and wrap it around his or her upper arms—above the elbows. The rope will want to slip if you don't have enough tension on it. **Tip:** Ask your sexy partner to push gently against the rope while you are putting the wraps on.

3. When the wraps are on, you will pass the rope around the middle, just like you did with the kneeling tie. Pick up the wraps on the other side and gently pull the arms together at the elbow and cinch it down. **Tip:** Not everyone's body can do this, and there is nothing wrong with that.

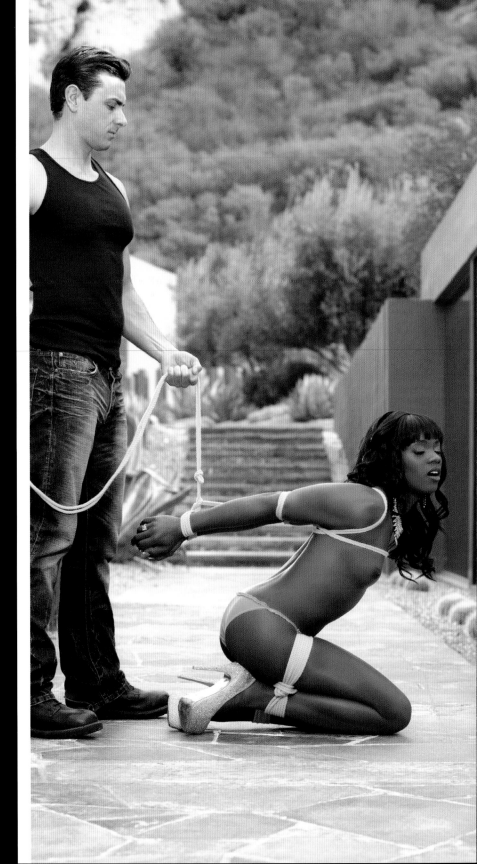

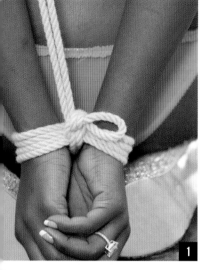

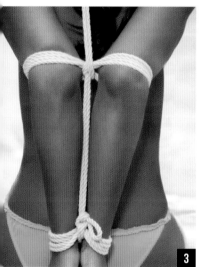

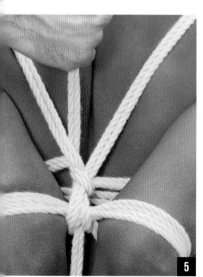

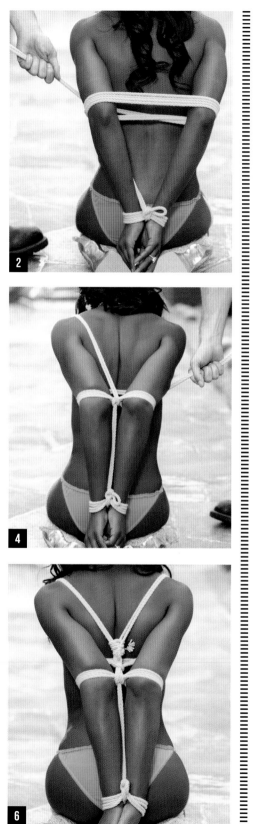

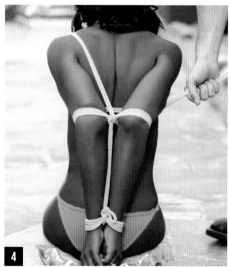

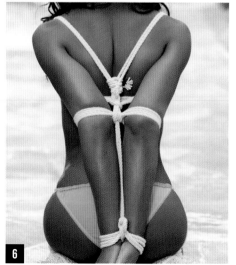

A way to help your body a bit is to raise your elbows upward; that pulls the elbows away from the body and gives more room for flexibility. Listen to your partner: You DON'T want to tie to the point of pain.

4. Take the rope and come over the left shoulder. Instead of crossing the chest, just drop the rope down and through the left armpit and bring it across the back. I know it is hard to see in this picture, but stay with me on this one—it is going to look awesome in a moment!

5. Come across the back, up through the right armpit, and over the right shoulder, and now back to the cinch where the elbows are deliciously trapped.

6. You should be almost out of rope. Finish the tie in a nice pretty way. Extra points if you make a bow!

FINAL: Now your partner is completely under your control! You can lift the arms gently.

Tip: Having your partner bend forward will let his or her arms come higher and make the position feel more submissive. Make sure to go slow and gently with this though; you want a sexy stretch, not a painful one.

MEN'S CHEST HARNESS

This is an intermediate chest tie that takes only one length of rope and a followed pattern to pull it together. This chest harness is designed to accentuate a masculine chest and keep your man's arms firmly behind his back where they belong when YOU are in charge!

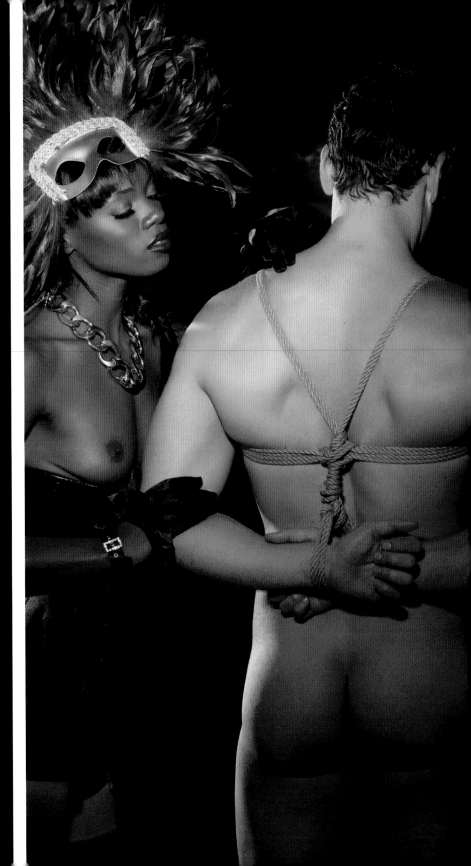

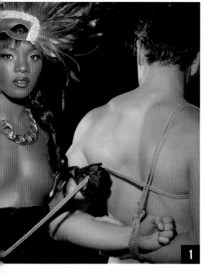

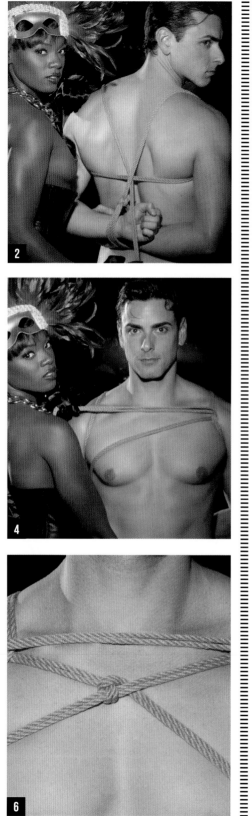

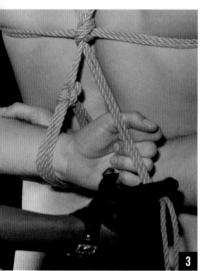

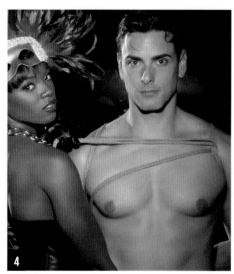

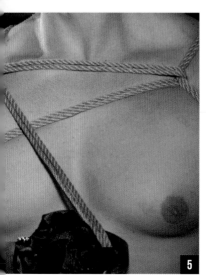

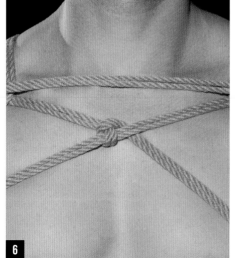

1. Capture the wrists using the Wrists Behind tie (page 96) and come up over the right shoulder, then down through the armpit to the back.

2. Come across the back, up through the left armpit and over the left shoulder, and then back to the center.

3. You don't even need a knot here, just a few wraps to keep it all in place.

4. Now, come up through the right armpit again, across the chest, and pull it through the left shoulder rope.

5. Come back and under the right shoulder rope. It should match this picture.

6. Form a quick Munter Hitch (page 90) and go across the chest and through the left armpit to the back and tie it off.

FINAL: Now that he's restrained so handsomely, its time to take control of his cock. It takes a strong man to be in this kind of rope!

BASIC FUTO

This is a very basic beginning to a great Futo tie (a Western name for a Japanese bondage standard). It is more complicated than the simple Two-Column Tie (page 98) but it looks very pretty and is for when you are ready to take the next step. It has the added bonus that the multiple wraps spread the tie out and make it much more comfortable than the Two-Column Tie. The knots run up and down both sides. This particular Futo has a very simple connecting of the horizontal wraps.

1. Start with a simple Bula Bula (page 86) or Sommerville Bowline (page 92) around the ankle.

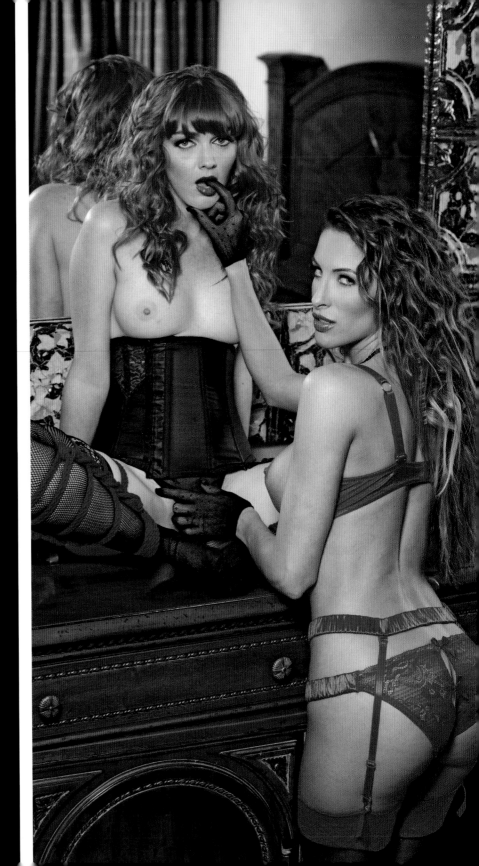

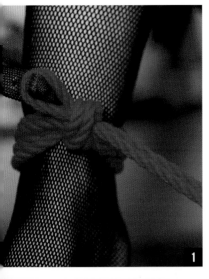

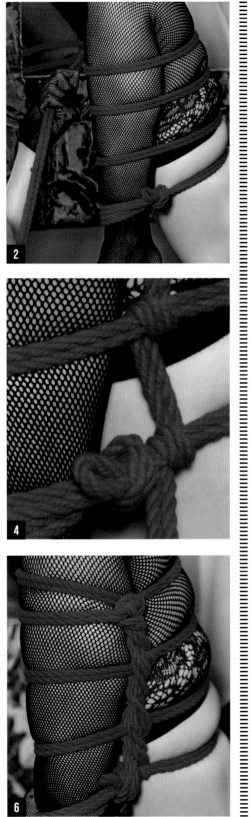

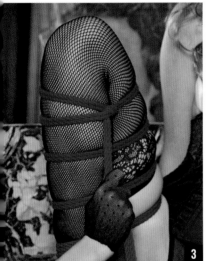

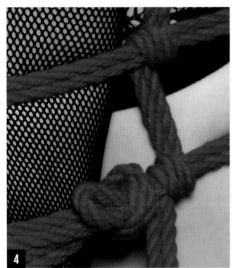

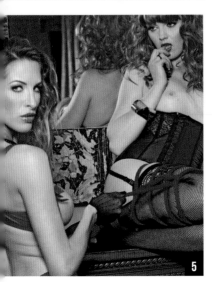

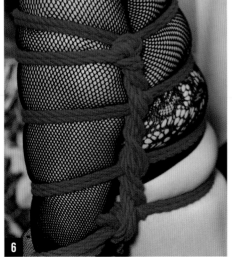

2. Wrap from the bottom upward, keeping the lower leg pushed against the thigh. This tie works best when the leg is tight to the body and the wraps start high on the thigh up near the hip joint.

3. Make four wraps, then when you come around the top, bring a final half wrap around to catch the top horizontal wrap, just like this.

4. Make a simple overhand wrap around each horizontal and work your way downward like this.

5. Once you reach the bottom and have it wrapped, tuck it under the last wrap and through. Then get your sexy rope bunny to bend her leg forward so you can do the same to the outside, working your way upward.

6. If you have a lot of rope left once you reach the top of the knee on the outside of the leg, retrace your steps, building a new layer over the top of what you just made, coming back through and back up the inside, wrapping in a twisting motion around all the verticals, just to make it pretty and keep the rope from getting tangled in the rest of your playtime.

FINAL: And what happens when you get them all tied up with their legs spread? I'm sure you can think of a few tasty things to do!

Now that we've mastered the arm binder, let's move on to the binding of the legs! This is a great tie to do when your lover is lying down.
It is safer than having him or her potentially fall over, and it's a great
tie for a rope bunny who likes to feel helpless and completely bound.

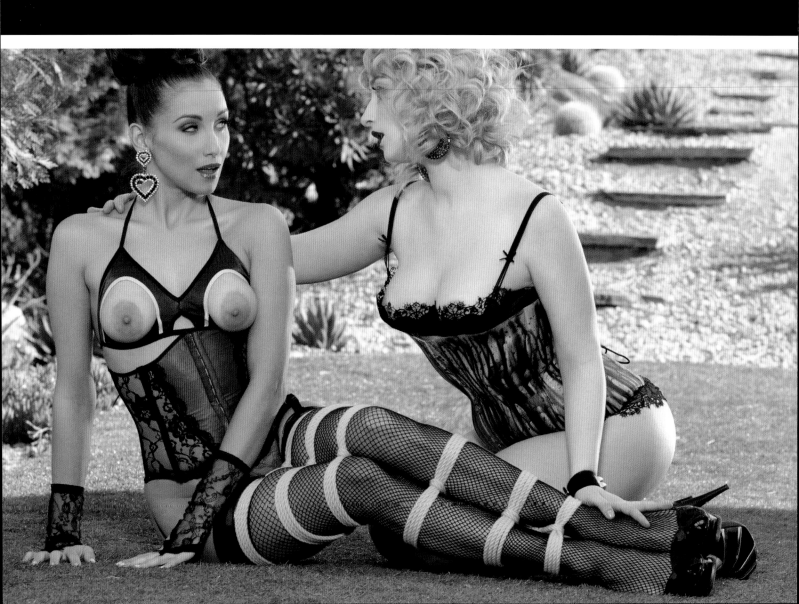

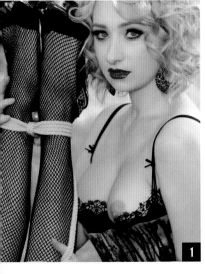
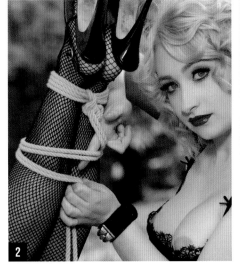
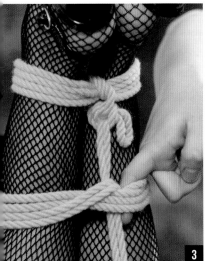
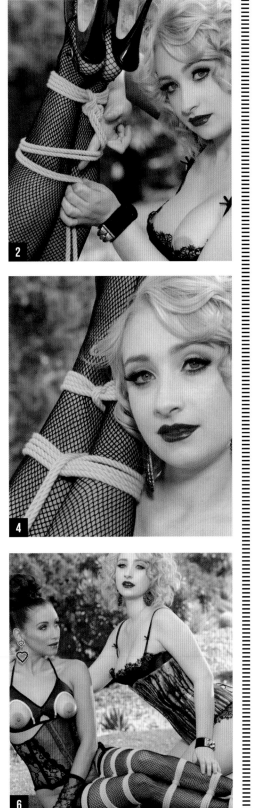
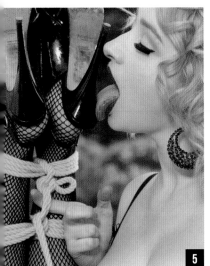
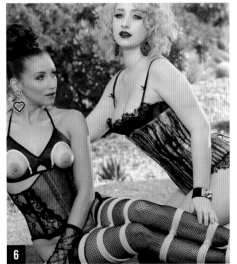

1. Here we see Allura with a simple Two-Column Tie (page 98) applied to Celeste's ankles.

2. Come around the back with the rope and make two wraps around the shins.

3. See how she tucks the rope up and over the wraps on the other side of the vertical rope?

4. You don't even have to tie a knot in the back if you can keep the tension on the rope. Come between the legs and up over the shin wraps.

5. Come back through and make a wrap around the vertical rope again.

6. Repeat all the way up the body, making wraps every 10 inches (25 cm). Tie just below and above the knees—not right on the joint.

FINAL: If you want, you can continue the tie all the way up the body! What a lovely way to spend a sunny afternoon on the lawn.

ASYMMETRIC CHEST TIE FOR MEN

This tie builds somewhat on the foundation of some of the earlier chest harnesses. It is also an asymmetrical tie, which means if you draw a line down the middle of Ryan, our bunny, each side looks different. It is fun, strong, and when tied over clothes that are later pulled open, looks super sexy. All the main knots are in the back rather than on the front.

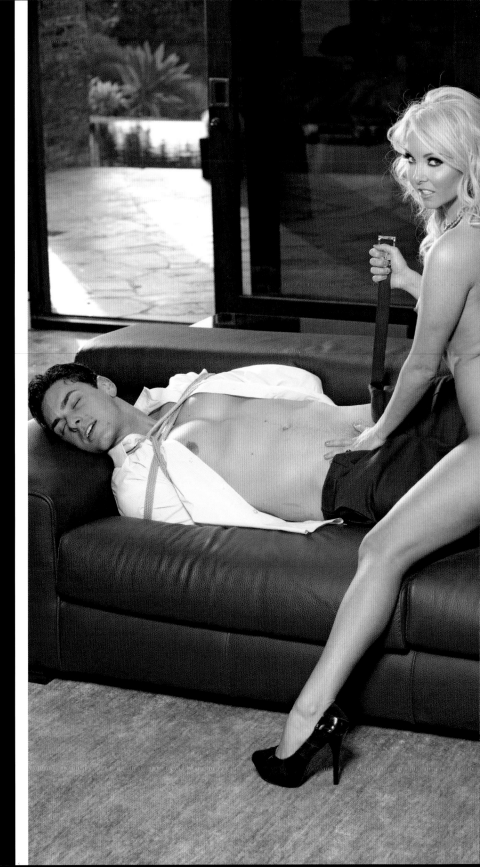

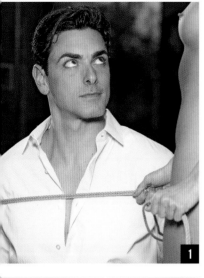

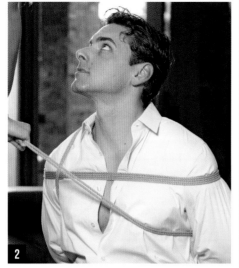

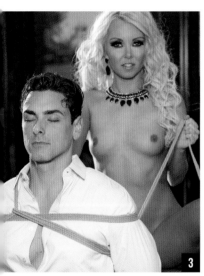

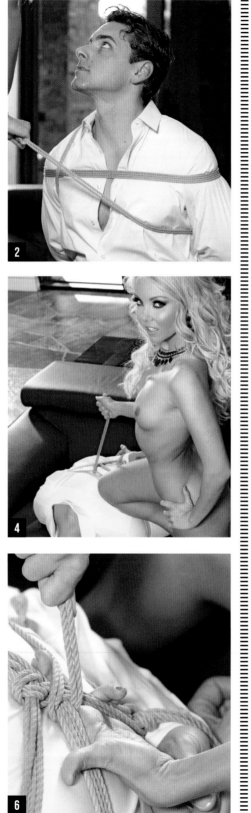

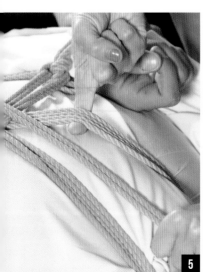

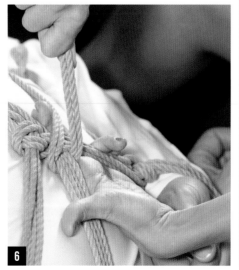

1. It all starts with his hands tied behind his back in a Two-Column Tie (page 98), then you start by wrapping his chest and shoulder, above his nipple line.

2. Get two wraps around the chest and shoulders and then, on the right-hand side, come up between his arm and chest and up over the shoulder. Then pull the rope down under his left armpit and across the front.

3. Go back the way you came. You should have a nice, neat set of wraps that look just like this, pulling on the vertical rope over his right shoulder.

4. Don't be afraid to show him who's boss. You're in charge! Bend him over and put your knee on him to hold him in place as you finish the ties in the back.

5. Carry the free end of the rope and pull up the lower wrap.

6. Tuck it under and cinch it tight, then finish with a knot in the back.

FINAL: Yes, that's right. Be a good boy and do everything the wicked lady tells you to!

SEXY SELF-TIED CHEST HARNESS

No one says you have to have your partner tie you up! You can make yourself pretty all by yourself. However, like the responsible adults we are, never do any type of bondage alone, including solo. Always have someone with you; it's good practice. Have a pair of safety scissors nearby. Here is Ana tying up her chest and those great, perky breasts!

1. She starts with a simple loop around her chest, underneath the breasts.

2. Come through the loop and reverse around the way you just came, back around the chest.

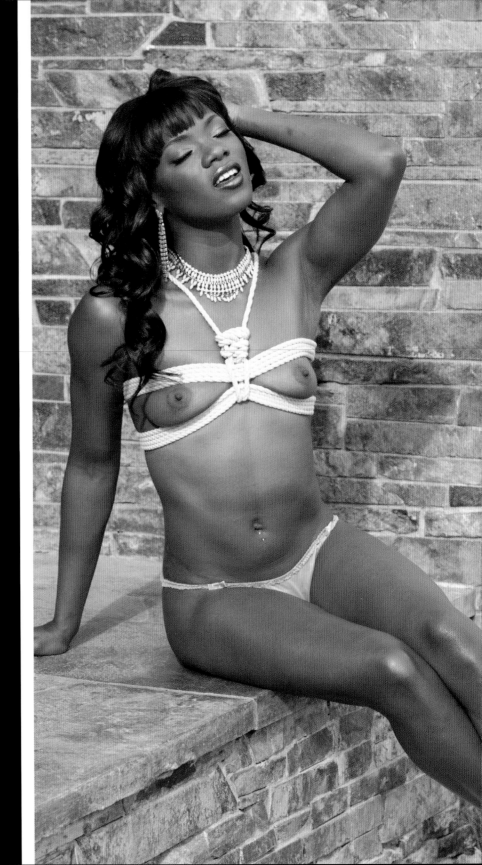

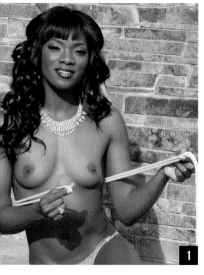

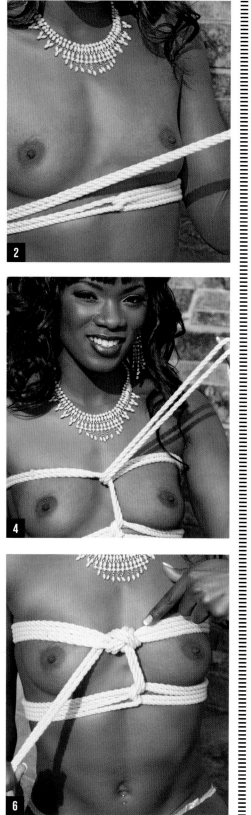

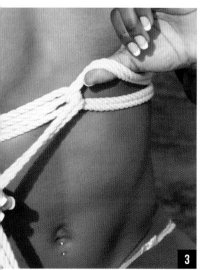

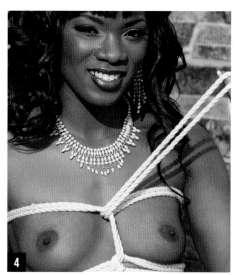

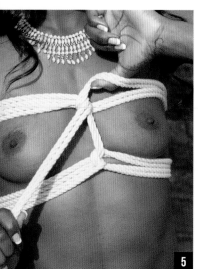

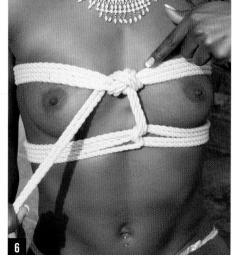

3. Look closely; see the original loop you created when you passed the rope back around the body? You are going to pull the rope through that loop.

4. Now take the rope straight up between the breasts, hold it in place while you change direction and make a wrap around the chest again, this time above the breasts. **Tip:** If you keep the tension on the rope as you do this, it makes it more manageable and stops it from falling off your body.

5. Just like the first wrap did a double pass around the chest down below, you are going to repeat the same step above the breasts. Pass it around and then come back through the loop you just created.

6. This is where you can get creative with tying it off. You can make a pair of diagonal passes with the rope. Then you can pass the rope around to the back of the body.

FINAL: We always like to use up the remaining 3 to 4 feet (91 to 122 cm) of rope in a creative way, and this is a perfect opportunity! Here, Ana has come up her shoulders and passed the rope down to the vertical rope in between her breasts and finished with a simple weaving back and forth to finish the ends. Use any variation you like; get creative!

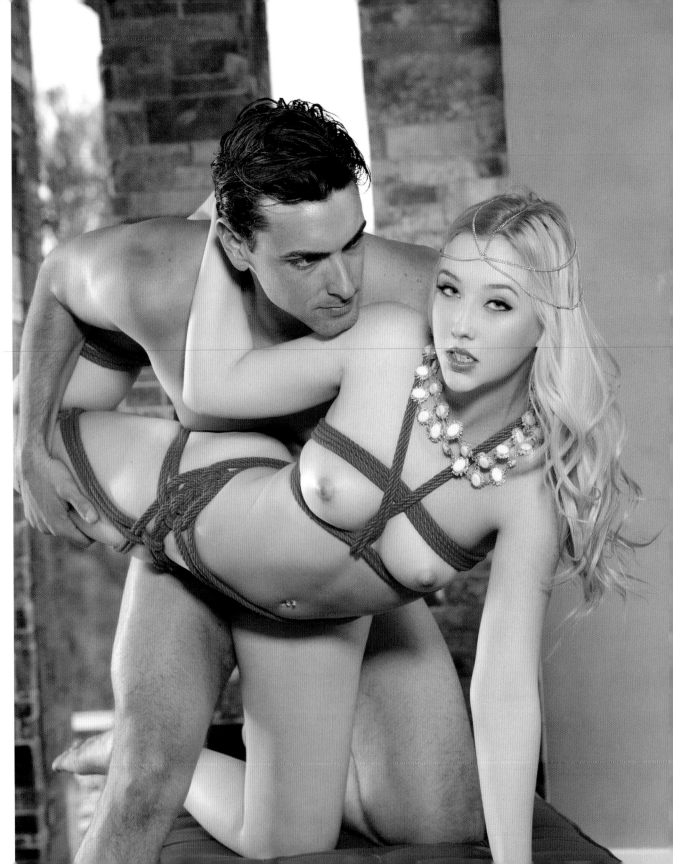

Chapter 8

TAKING IT FURTHER

By now, you should be feeling a lot more confident wielding a nice bit of rope. You should be thinking, talking, and dreaming about nothing but rope. You might be asking yourself how you can progress from these basic ties. One of the best things about the world of rope bondage is that you never stop learning. Now you can piece together your knowledge of the basics to form intermediate ties and create new, delicious works of art. In this chapter, you'll see how some binds can be extended to form full-torso harnesses or to allow you to tie arms and legs together at the same time. You'll see that basically all the more intermediate ties are built upon the same foundations that we practiced in chapter 6; from these basics, a multitude of different variations can be made.

There's nothing more scintillating than binding your sub(s) in beautifully intricate arrangements, feeling her pulse quicken beneath the warmth of your palm, and seeing her eyes silently beg you for more. These harnesses are perfect for having your filthy way with someone.

FINGER TIE

Tying up the body is great fun, but many people don't think about making their partners sensually helpless by tying their fingers and toes. And as a bonus, it is great fun in a bubble bath. Here Sophia is using colored thick acrylic yarn from the craft store to tie up Spencer's fingers in microbondage. A man-made fiber won't shrink or lose its color when it is wet. Fingers are delicate and we don't want the binding material to constrict. The best part is it is so cheap that when you are done you just snip it off and toss it in the garbage, which makes for easy clean-up.

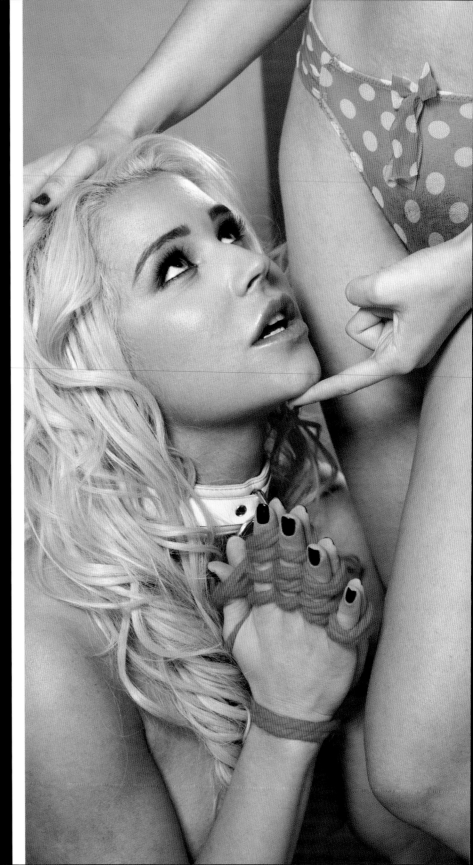

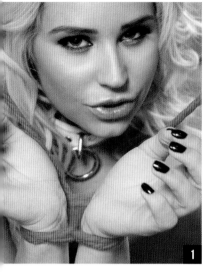

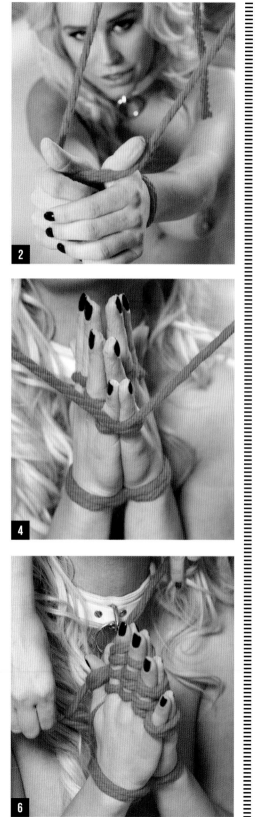

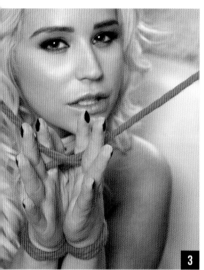

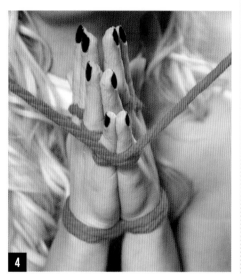

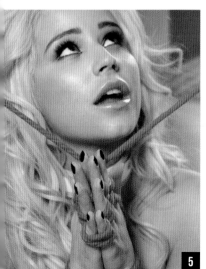

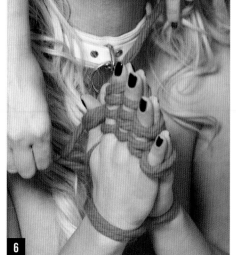

1. Wrap a Lark's Head (page 88) around the wrist and then come back through the middle, the same as all the other two-column ties in the book.

2. Split the ends and come around the thumbs. Make the yarn snug but not so tight that it cuts off the circulation. You want your pet to be tied enough to be comfortable but not so much that their fingernails turn blue.

3. After you come around the thumbs, have her spread her fingers and start to weave back and forth between the fingers.

4. Work all the way down until you get to the end and cross around the pinkies.

5. Adjust the tension as needed.

6. Work your way back to the thumbs, going back the way you came and tie back between the thumbs or the wrists, whichever you can reach comfortably

FINAL: Now she is all pretty and captured. What you do next is up to your imagination.

TOE TIE

Would you believe me if I told you there is a tie that will allow you to delay or deny your partner's orgasm? If you notice your partner when they are having an orgasm, check to see if they point or flex their toes. Eighty percent of people will point. If you tie the foot and toes in the opposite direction, it will make it incredibly difficult for them to orgasm, or that is to say they can orgasm when *you* want them to.

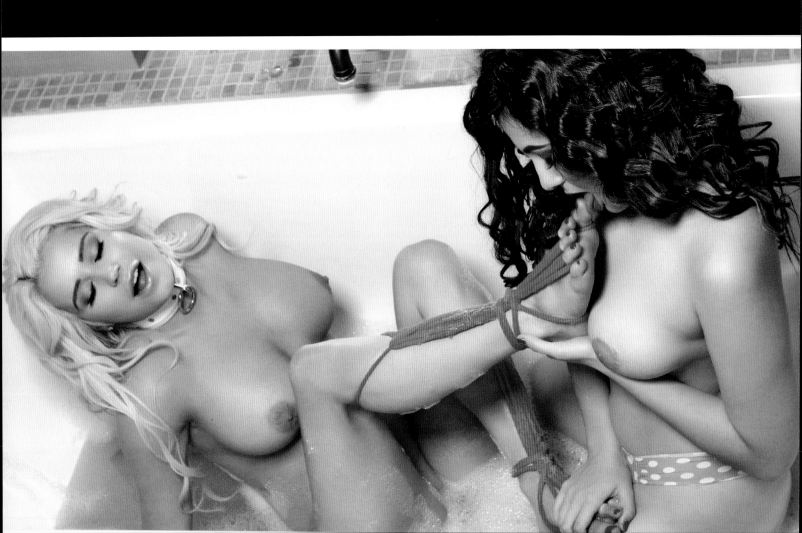

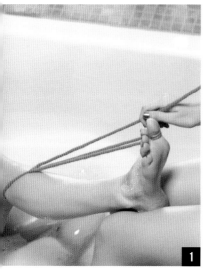
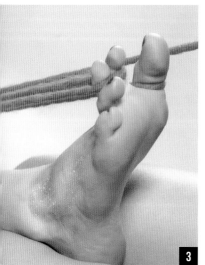
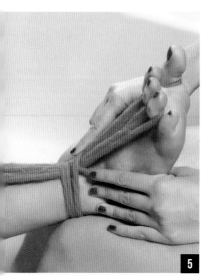
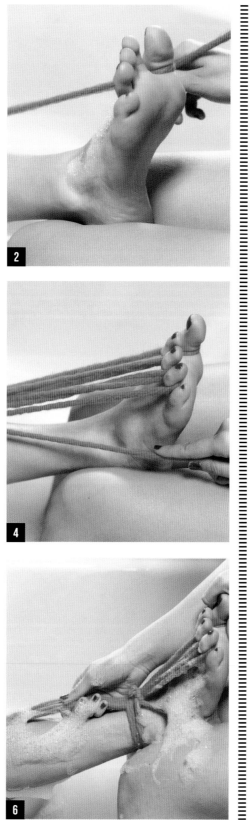
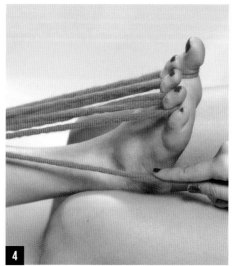
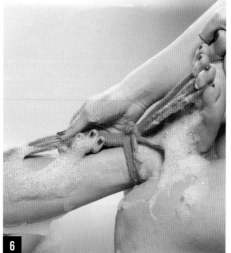

1. First, start with a tie under the knee but above the calf. You want the bulge of the calf to hold this loop in place. It doesn't have to be tight as you will need to be able to slip a few fingers through it. Next come down to the big toe and make a wrap and then return to the calf loop, making this part snug.

2. In this close-up, notice that the width of the yarn is still comfortable for the toe.

3. Repeat: Come down from the calf loop to the second toe and return, then the do the same for the third toe.

4. Continue all the way until you get to the fourth toe. We normally don't tie the last toe.

5. Come back with the yarn to the ankle and make a big wrap around the ankle, pulling the strands into one bundle. This is how you fine-tune the tie and make it exactly as tight as you want.

6. It also makes a handy handle!

FINAL: Tie both feet and have at it. For safety's sake, your tied partner should stay reclining. The water is warm, the feet are tied, and you can take her to the edge of orgasm without worrying about her falling over. Enjoy!

SIMPLE AND SEXY CHEST HARNESS FOR WOMEN

This is a great, simple chest harness to start with, as it will act as a foundation for adding to the bondage later on. It's fun and makes breasts stand up just a little more, leaving them aching to be caressed. Chest harnesses form a foundation in rope bondage as a point to stand on their own or as the start of something more complex, which we will see later in the book.

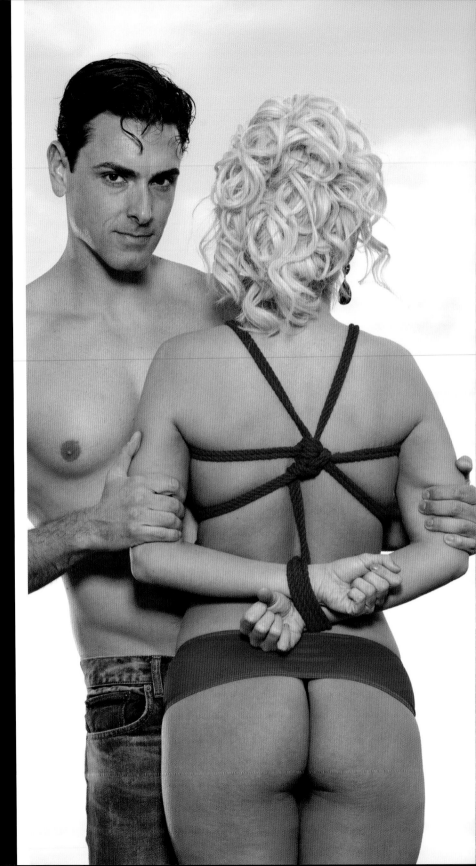

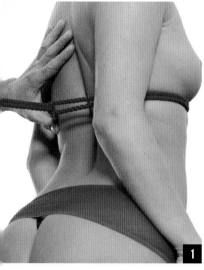

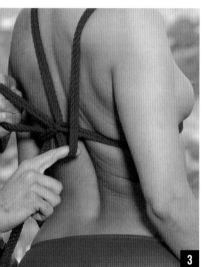

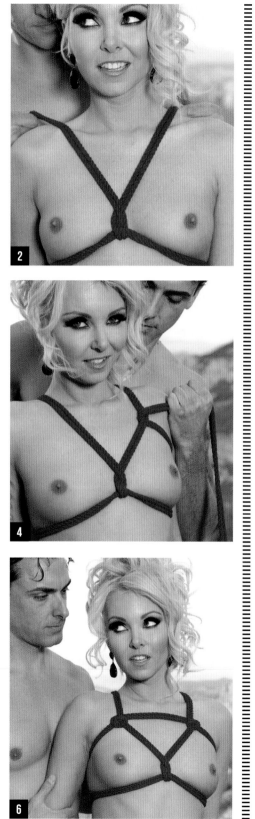

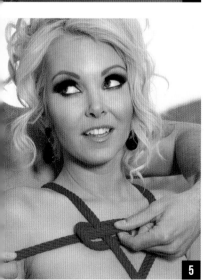

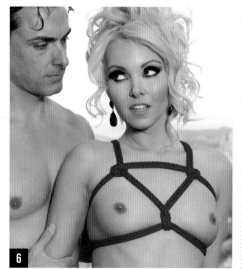

1. Begin by pulling the rope around the body and back through the loop, or bight, which is the middle of the rope.

2. Come up and over the shoulder and down to the middle, crossing over and under, then back up again over the opposite shoulder.

3. Pull the rope over the right shoulder and bring it up and under the horizontal wrap. Pull it up between the wrap and the base of the left shoulder rope and make a simple knot to hold it secure.

4. Come around the front, under the arm, and pull the rope from under and then inside to out. You are going to form a Munter Hitch (page 90) here.

5. See? Just like this from one rope to the other.

6. Looking beautiful!

FINAL: After you have tied it off in the back, if you have any left over, drop a length down and bundle up your partner's wrists. Your bunny will be extra captive!

WRIST CAPTURE

This is a fun variation on the previous tie, taking it to a whole new level!

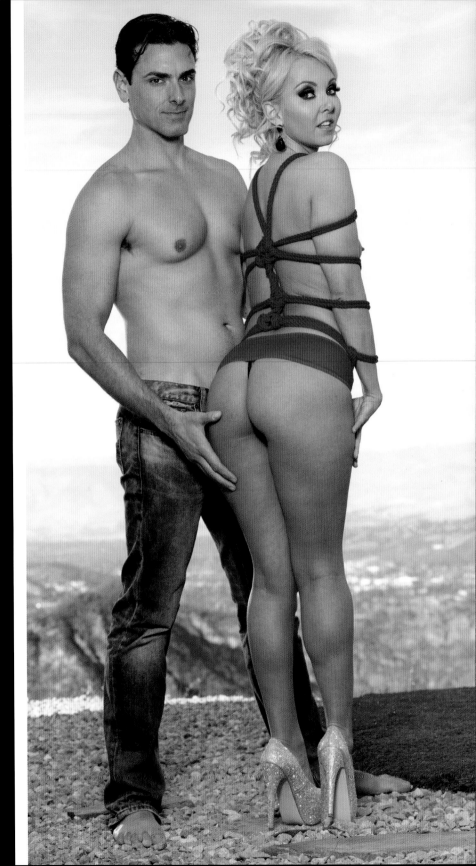

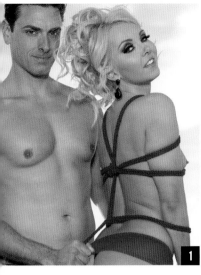

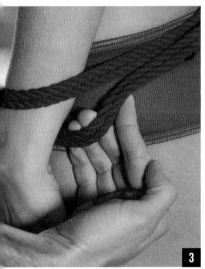

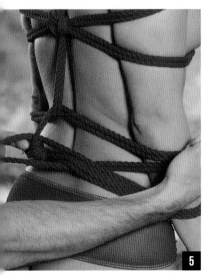

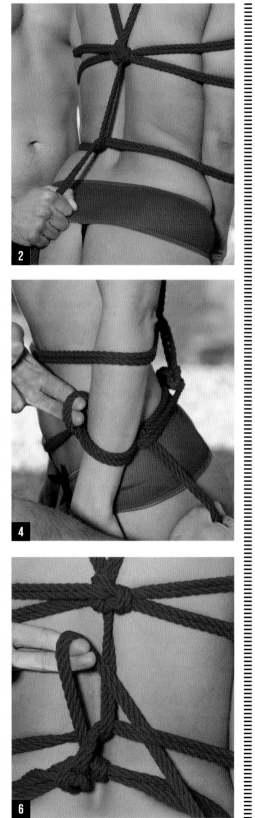

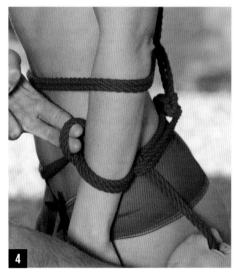

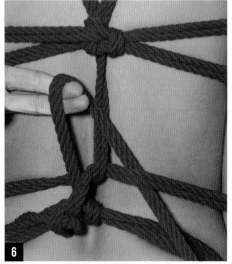

1. If you want to take the chest harness a little further, don't tie her hands behind her back. Have them relax at her sides and put another loop around them down lower, trapping the arms just above the wrists.

2. Bring the rope around through the rope running down the middle of her back, then come back the way you came.

3. Come back to the wrist and feed the rope on the inside of the wrist.

4. Bring it up and around and back through the way you just came, cinching the wrists snugly. Then go back around and do the other wrist.

5. Come back around the rope, down the spine, and make a loop around it.

6. Knot it all off in the back and make it nice and neat. Neatness counts for great rope bondage; you don't want to be sloppy!

FINAL: She's now snug and secure and ready for a spanking!

NOVICE CHEST HARNESS

Here's a chest harness that is the next step up in complexity but still easy enough to make sexy. It is a great way to accentuate the breasts and gain control over your sub's upper body.

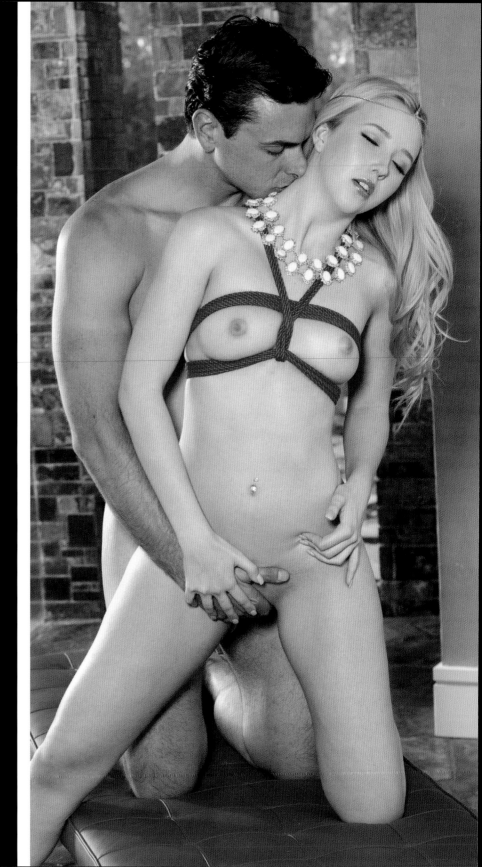

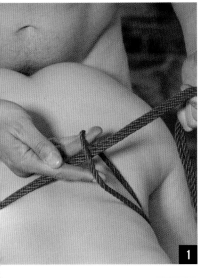

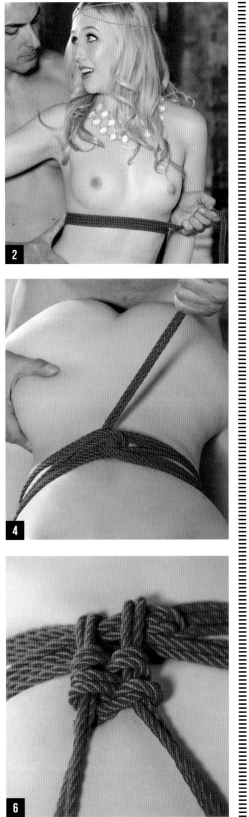

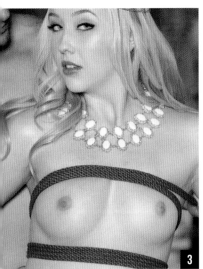

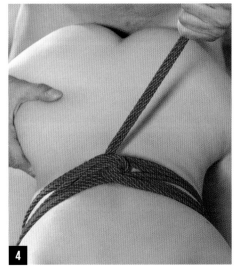

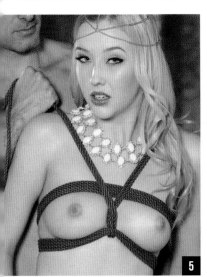

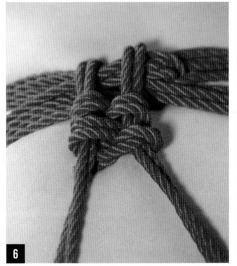

1. Start with a Lark's Head knot (page 88) around her rib cage.

2. Then wrap around the ribs right below the breasts. Do this twice.

3. Then make two wraps above the breasts.

4. Now pull the free end through the loops you made earlier. You've done this before.

5. Go over the shoulder and down between the breasts, picking up the lower wraps, and then give an extra twist as you come back up over the right shoulder.

6. When you come to the back, you can tie it off and take the leftover rope to weave it back and forth up the shoulder ropes you just made. It looks neat and sexy this way.

FINAL: Now that her top half is bound in your rope, use it as a harness to grab on to and have your way with her!

SIMPLE HIP HARNESS AND LEG WEAVE

This tie is more complex but not too hard and looks supersexy. Plus it acts as a sex harness, and we all like that, don't we?

1. Now that her chest and breasts are bound, its time to control her bottom half too. Get her up against the wall and start with a Lark's Head knot (page 88) around the waist.

2. Wrap around the waist twice and then make a half hitch on the hip, just like you see here.

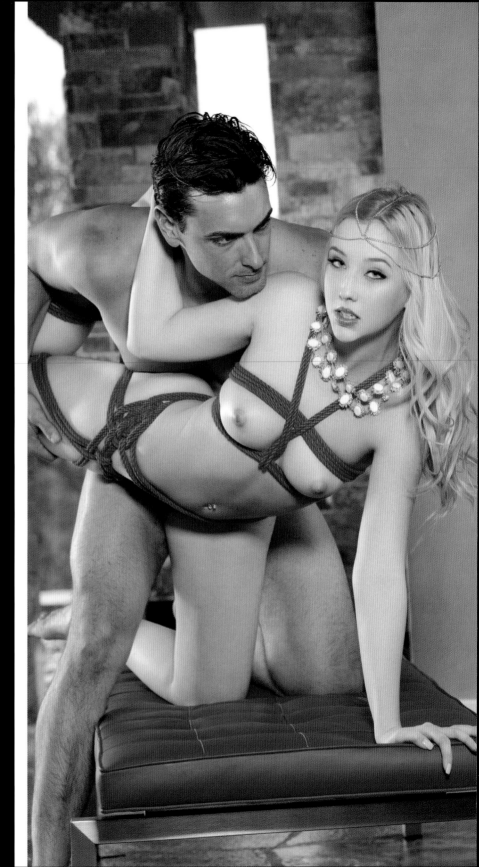

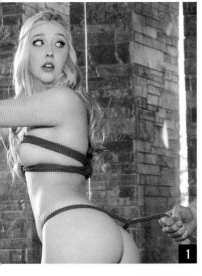

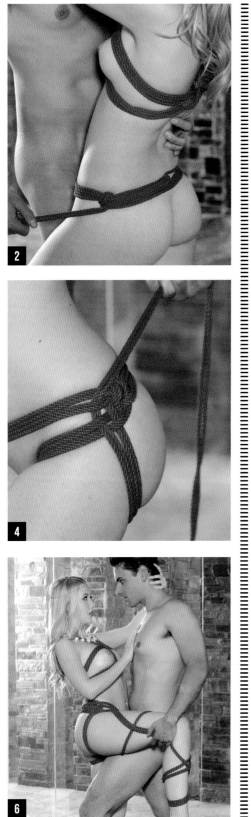

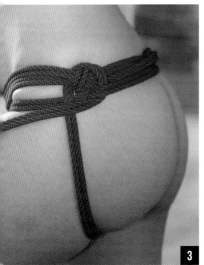

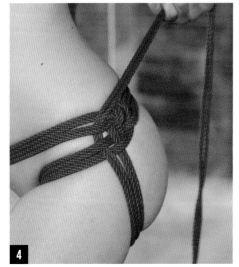

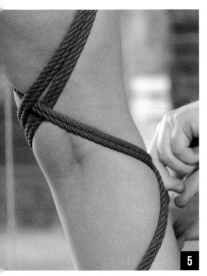

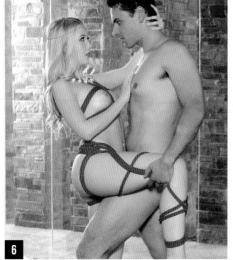

3. Stay with me on this one—it is about to get intense and sexy! Bring the rope across the front of her thigh, down between her legs, and up in the crease of her bum, all the way up to the original hitch on the side. Go OVER the wrap you just made and UNDER the waist wraps and then OVER the next part of the waist and then UNDER the one you just brought up from the crease of the ass. Isn't that looking pretty now?

4. Repeat, following the same path, making the opposite weave right beside the line you are following. The more you build, the sexier it gets!

5. Once you get the waist harness looking the way you want, you can use another length of rope and start winding down and around the thigh and leg. Remembering to weave opposite as you trace back through.

6. Ooooooh! Things are getting steamy! All these ropes make for great grab points during sex.

FINAL: Like this one! This tie makes a great handle for from-behind-sex. Use it to pull your partner in close and keep her there!

NOVICE SEX HARNESS HIP TIE

Want more control during sex? This hip harness provides multiple leverage points to get your partner exactly where you want him or her. The great thing about this tie is that it uses the great weaving technique we love, which makes the knots minimal, and that makes it very comfortable. It also leaves the pussy and ass open for all sorts of fun.

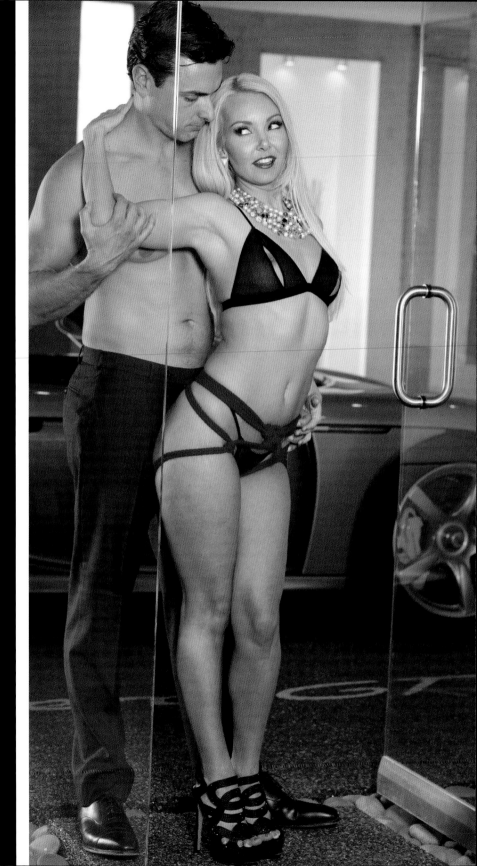

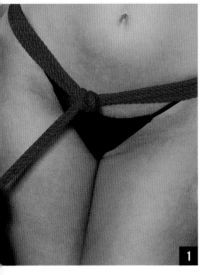
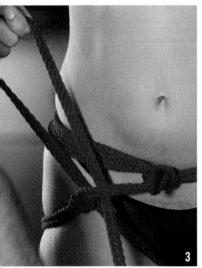
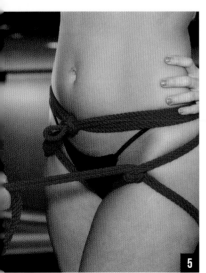
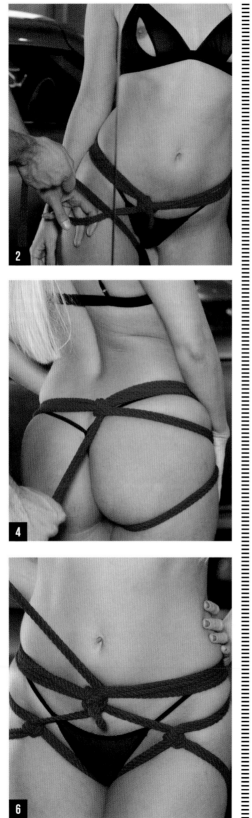
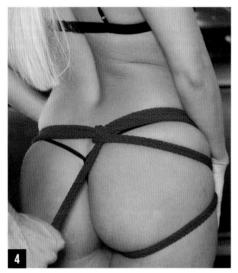
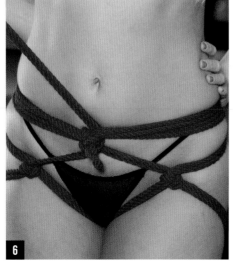

1. Start with a simple hip wrap going twice around the body and finishing with a Bula Bula (page 86) or a Sommerville Bowline (page 92) right in the front.

2. Come over the thigh, under the bum, and up between the legs.

3. Meet that thigh rope with a quick and easy Munter Hitch (page 90) and pull through.

4. Bring that rope around the back and make a quick hitch to keep the rope up high off that tasty ass; you don't want it falling down and getting in the way of sexy time!

5. Pull it around to the front, down between the legs, and up over the ass, and meet that first rope with another Munter Hitch.

6. Take the free end and pull it up into the knot in the middle of the waist wrap; cross over and up.

FINAL: Now pull on those ropes for leverage while thrusting and really make your partner scream with pleasure!

THE INFINITY

Now that you have something to grab on to, let's create another tie that uses simple weaving to accentuate the breasts. Big or small, it does it all!

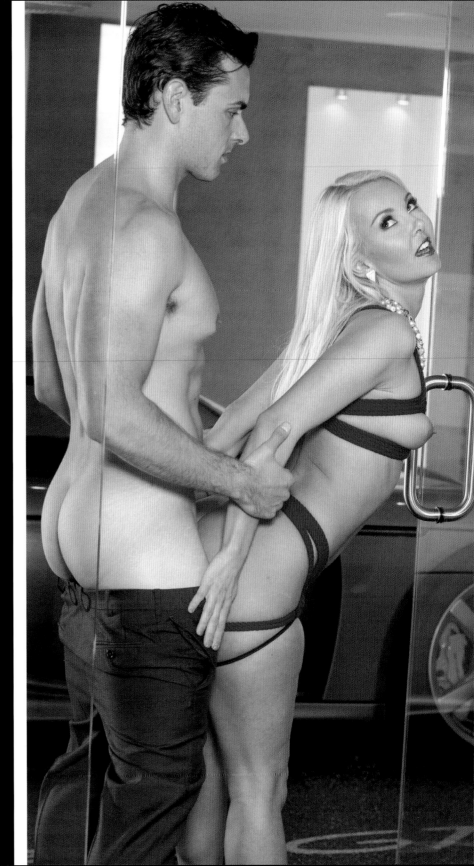

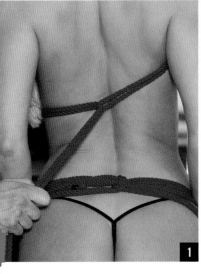

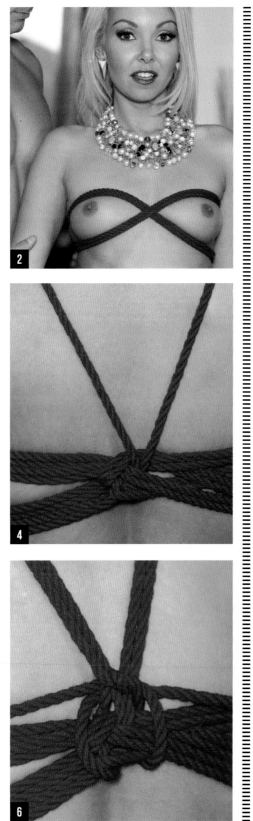

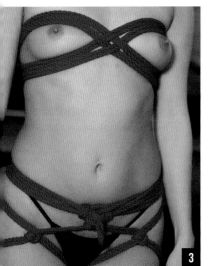

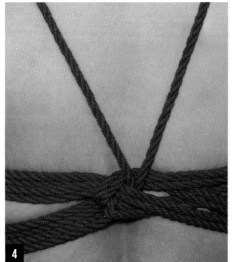

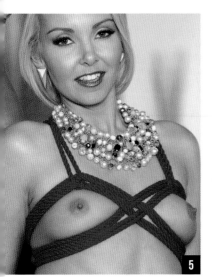

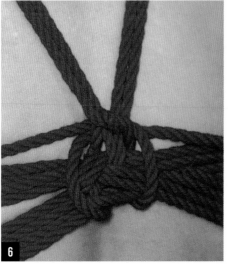

1. Put a wrap around the chest, this time coming up and over one breast.

2. Now change direction. Come around the front and go up and over the other breast.

3. Repeat, building on the last. Isn't this fun and pretty? Weave in and out as you cross over each new wrap.

4. Keep the back nice and neat, and when you have about 3 feet (0.91 m) left of rope, split the pair in your hand and come up and over the shoulders and over to the front.

5. Weave it down into the top wraps. This will keep it from falling as you get into the hardcore fun times.

6. Try to keep it neat when you come back to the original knot. You can even use a bow if you like.

FINAL: Time to admire those lovely breasts from behind! Don't get too distracted . . .

SEXY BODY TIE OR KARADA

This tie uses a series of knots to form attractive diamond patterns across the body, typically known as a *Karada* in the west. It is a great way to decorate your partner and make your bunny feel as attractive as we know he or she is!

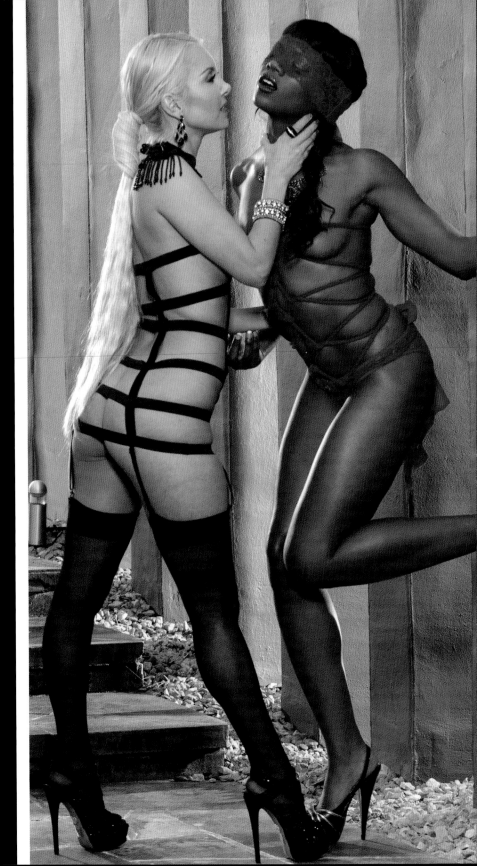

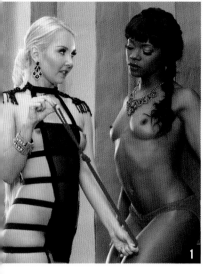

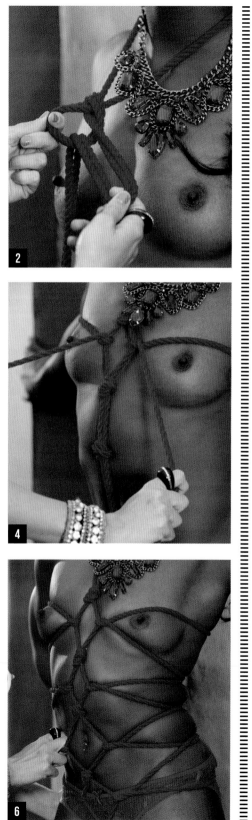

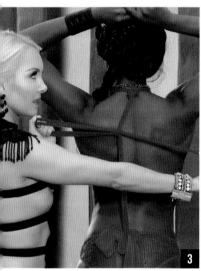

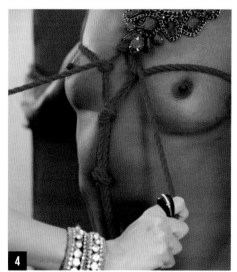

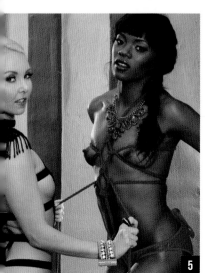

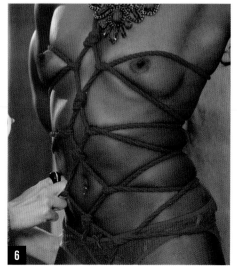

1. Aayliah starts with tying a simple overhand knot about a foot down in the rope at the bight end.

2. Slip it over your partner's head so the knot you just made sits on the back of their neck. Create a new knot between the collarbone and nipples.

3. Make a series of knots about 6 inches (15 cm) apart all the way down as you bring the rope between the legs and up the back, pulling the ends through the first loop that is hanging down your partner's back.

4. Now is the time for the splits! Because we tie with doubled-over rope, we can separate it at any time and go in different directions. Just like now: Come under the arms and pull the rope through the vertical rope between each knot and then go back the way you came, opening up the diamond in the process.

5. Wrap around the back and come back to make the next diamond.

6. Come all the way down the body. Doesn't she look tasty?

FINAL: Transforming your slave into a walking work of art can be extremely rewarding. Now it's time to admire!

ASS OPENER

We have already seen a nice, easy, self-tying chest harness earlier in the book. This is a perfect tie for the bottom half of a woman where she can play with herself or use it as a completely fuckable tie for anal and vibrator stimulation! Samantha is going to show you how.

1. Start with a few wraps around the body—you have seen this before and are a pro at it by now. This time end the wraps in the front.

2. Make a nice simple knot around the whole series of wraps and tighten it.

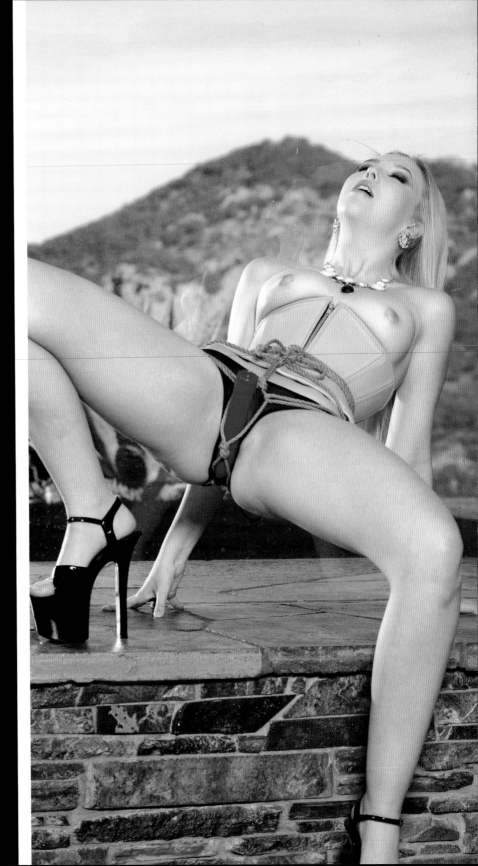

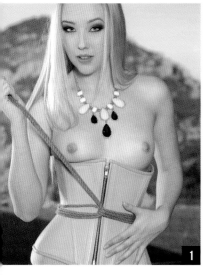

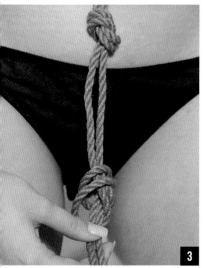

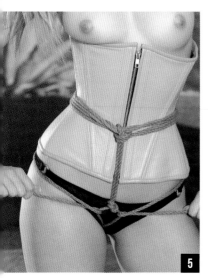

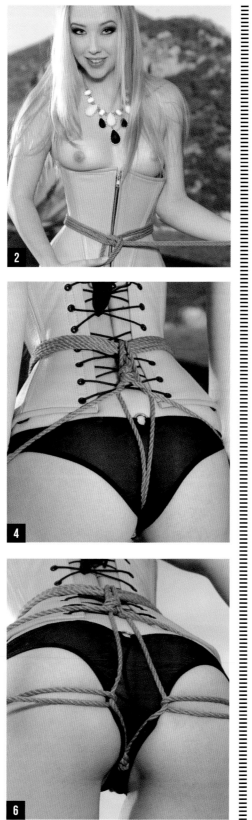

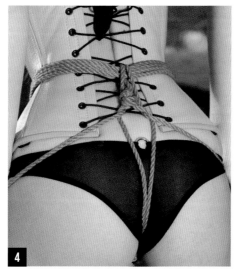

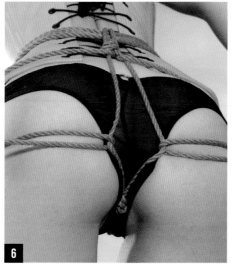

3. Now you are going to make two knots down the rope as it hangs in front of the pussy. The lower knot should hang either right in front of the clit or just below it.

4. Samantha turns around and pulls the rope up and through the waist wraps and makes a knot. Now can you see how she pulls the ends and the back is starting to open up? To ease into anal sex, it takes just another step or two.

5. First, she is going to come around the front with each end and pull through the doubled rope across the pussy and tug the lips open with rope. Yummy.

6. Then she passes the ropes around the back and splits apart the back part of the rope, tying it off in the front around the waist and now she is all ready for some anal play and more!

FINAL: Who says you can't have a hands-free orgasm?!

REDNECK TRUCKER'S HITCH

Yee-haw! This is the sexiest version of the Redneck Trucker's Hitch. Y'all are going to rope your little filly into a classic spread-eagle tie to the bed. This tie uses a special hitch so no matter how much of a sexy struggle they put up, you can retighten them at any time, quickly.

1. Start with a Bula Bula (page 86) around the ankle.

2. Then make a slipknot just below the toe of the foot and go around a bedpost.

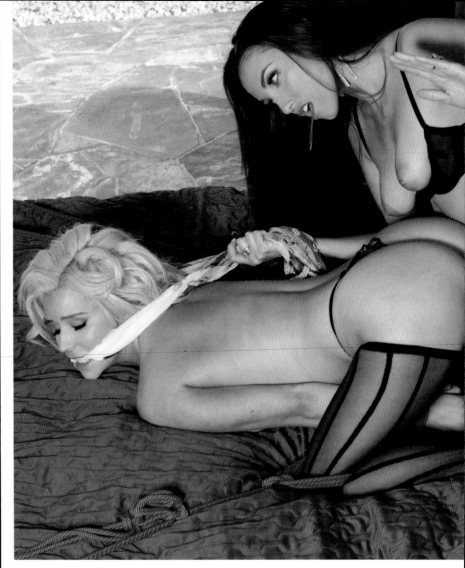

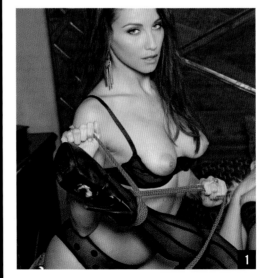

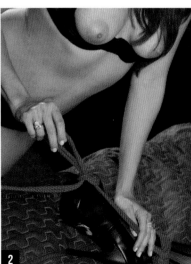

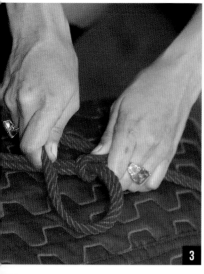

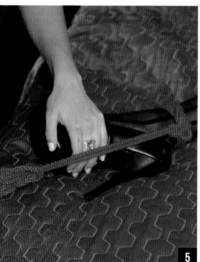

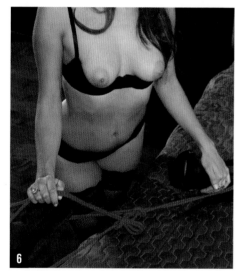

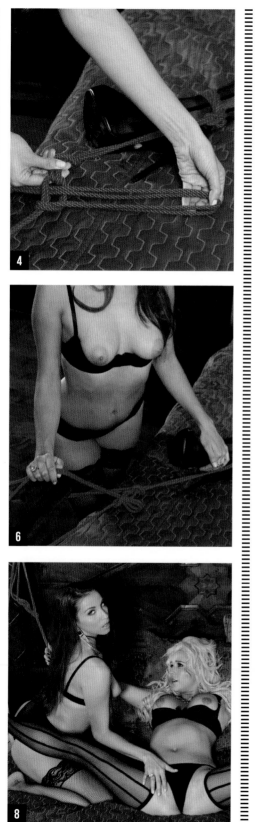

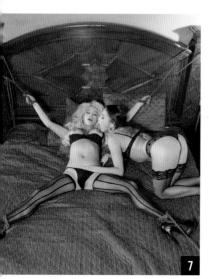

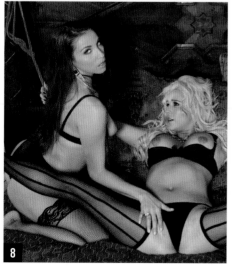

3. Stay with me here, almost done: Come around the bedpost with the free end and feed the loose end of the rope through the loop you just made and pull the leg snug. The loop will act just like a pully, then pinch the first loop to hold it in place for the next step, which is to make a loop just below it.

4. Pull a 12-inch (30 cm) loop through.

5. Snug it all up.

6. Now what you have is a slipknot that you can quickly pull the loose end of to free your partner—or if things get really steamy, to retighten the rope during sex. I like to call it "on-the-fly fucking."

7. Do this to all her arms and legs, and you can have her helpless in your power. Let's get 'er done!

8. You don't have to stick to the classic flat-on-the-back spreadeagle position. This tie is just as comfortable with legs up in the air, attached to the headboard posts.

FINAL: And here is the same tie attached to the thighs with Spencer facedown and ass up, ready for action! There are a lot of positions possible with this simple technique.

ROPE CORSET

Rope isn't just used to bind breasts in a chest tie. You can make a whole corset if you have enough rope. This tie is very straightforward: Once you get the first few wraps, the rest is easily repeated and your lover will look very tasty for you!

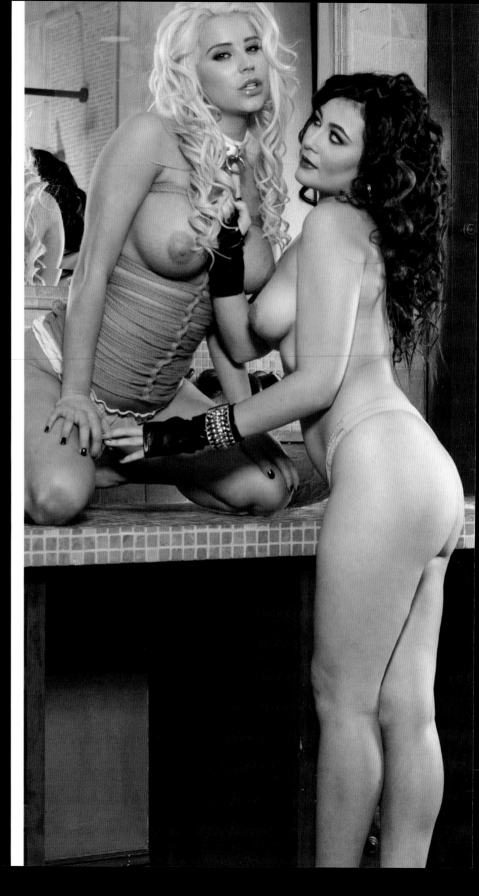

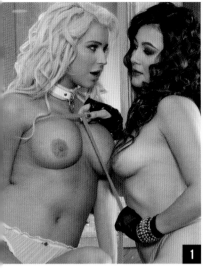

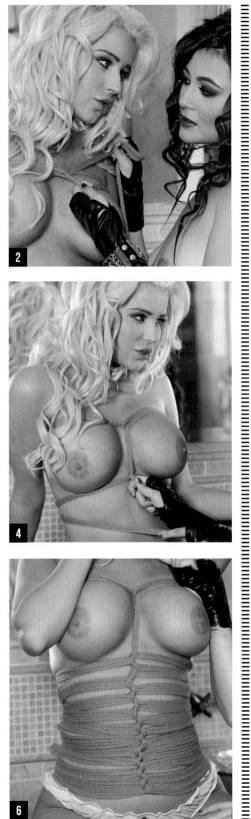

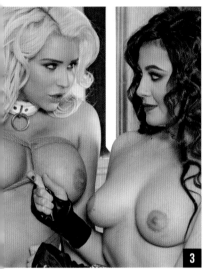

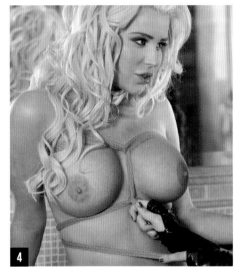

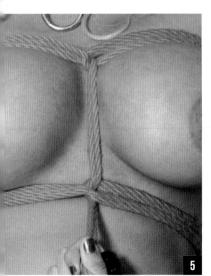

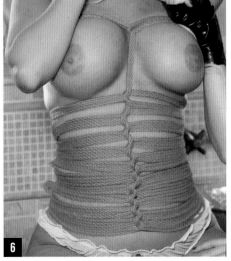

1. Start by capturing a loop around the back and pulling it to the front, keeping it above the breasts.

2. Feed the loose end through the loop and take a moment to admire your woman.

3. Bring the rope straight down between the breasts and hold it there while you come around the back to the front again.

4. Pass the loose end through the vertical rope and come right around the back again, making a full wrap.

5. Now come through the loop in the front, reverse the way you came, and . . .

6. . . . build it all the way down by simply repeating the same pattern over and over. When you run out of rope, just add more with the simple way to attach it shown on page 94.

FINAL: Now your girl is pretty enough to nibble on!

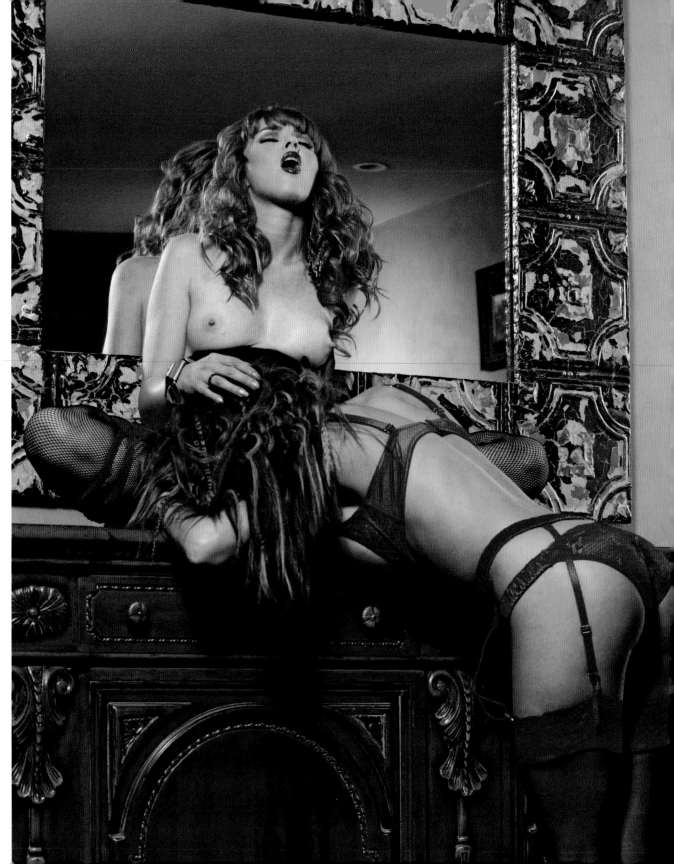

Chapter 9

WHAT'S NEXT?

Well done, you! Not only have you had the wisdom and foresight to buy this fantastic and alluring book, but you've also taken your first steps into bondage. By now, you're well versed in the basic chest harness and Two-Column Tie and have even pulled off a few leg ties as well. You've got your top-bottom communication down to a tee, and your toy box now contains EMT shears, bondage tape, blankets for aftercare, and some emergency dark chocolate with pistachios (good choice), as well as some quality rope. Congratulations! You're on your way to becoming a fantastic and inspiring rigger or a committed and exciting rope

WHERE TO GO FROM HERE

Well, there are dozens of avenues now open to you. Choice is overwhelming, as we all know, so ask yourself this question: What do you love most about bondage? Do you love the feeling of being restricted, whether it's being tied to a bedframe by your ankles or woven into gorgeous rope so you can't even wriggle an inch? Do you love the artistic flow that you feel when you have some tasty little sub under your knots, and you can use him or her as a canvas for your beautiful expression? Do you love being spanked while you're immobile, or tickled into submission by your caring, trustworthy top? Is it the possibility of giving your liberty over to the hands of a number of different dominant people that gets you hot under the collar? Or are you one of those sadistic devils who just loves to see a writhing rope bunny struggle beneath your ties?

Identifying your specific kink can open up a whole world of gorgeously sexy options to you if you feel that you'd like to explore bondage or BDSM even further. If, for instance, you feel confident that being a submissive is something you'd like to do more of, and your partner is practically bursting at the seams with the need to tie you up and ravish you, then perfect! You're lucky in that your kinks complement each other, and you've already got a partner who you trust implicitly. Sit down together, be honest about your fantasies and desires, and set about trying them. Can you think of a better way to spend a rainy Friday night?

However, if you're really into topping and love the idea of getting a whole range of tantalizing submissives under your rope, then you might want to think about getting out into your local kink community and finding some new willing partners to play with. Rope bondage is a craft like any other, and the more you practice, the better you will become. Remember those wise words from Picasso? "Learn the rules like a pro so you can break them like an artist." Perfect the building blocks outlined in this book and then find your own rope bondage style by combining the basics into something new and fresh. This is how I made my way to what I think of as my personal style today, and every single bunny who I get to play with teaches me something new, regardless if that person is experienced or new to rope bondage. There are a number of great books that will help you to be a better rigger, and you can find some of these listed in the resources section. Practice makes perfect—and why wouldn't you want to practice every day when your craft is as sensual as this?

EXPLORING ROPE FURTHER

Let's say that you've devoured all the information in this book a few times, salivated over the luscious photos, and have nearly worn the damn thing out by practicing the ties and checking on the suggestions for communication before and after playtime. Who can blame you? I can barely tear myself away from this thing, and I wrote it. You might have a dirty mind, but you have great taste!

There are many ways to move forward with rope. You'll most likely want to hone your skills, and though there are many fantastic books teaching intermediate bondage, there are also a large number of real-life classes in big cities around the globe. If you find a good, reputable teacher who has good standing in your local community, you will find these classes a great place to flourish in your craft, and they'll also provide wonderful opportunities to meet people who also love bondage and want to go further into the bondage world. Events like Shibaricon are world-renowned, and there are many smaller events in the same vein, so your opportunities for education and growth will be numerous.

You may even decide, eventually, that you want to become a bondage performer. The modern bondage community is as expansive as it is exciting, and there are bondage-themed events all over the world. In Toronto, Morpheous' Bondage Extravaganza has grown over eight years to become the world's largest public rope bondage event. This event, the highlight of my calendar, is a twelve-hour spree of rope-related revelry, with bunnies and riggers from all over the world showcasing their skills to thousands of visitors and viewers online, and all for free. It is a way to make the art of rope accessible for everyone without barriers. Though the riggers involved have many different styles, the diverse nature of the event means that we can showcase the very best of bondage for both art and sex, meaning that even the vanilla voyeurs who wander in accidentally end up staying all night. If your goal is to one day be a rigger up there on the stage making the audience gasp with pleasure, then seek out bondage events and immerse yourself in the community. You'll find mentors, bunnies, fans, and professionals there, and along with all these types of people comes opportunity. And I can't say it loud enough: Practice, practice, practice. These bunnies aren't going to tie themselves!

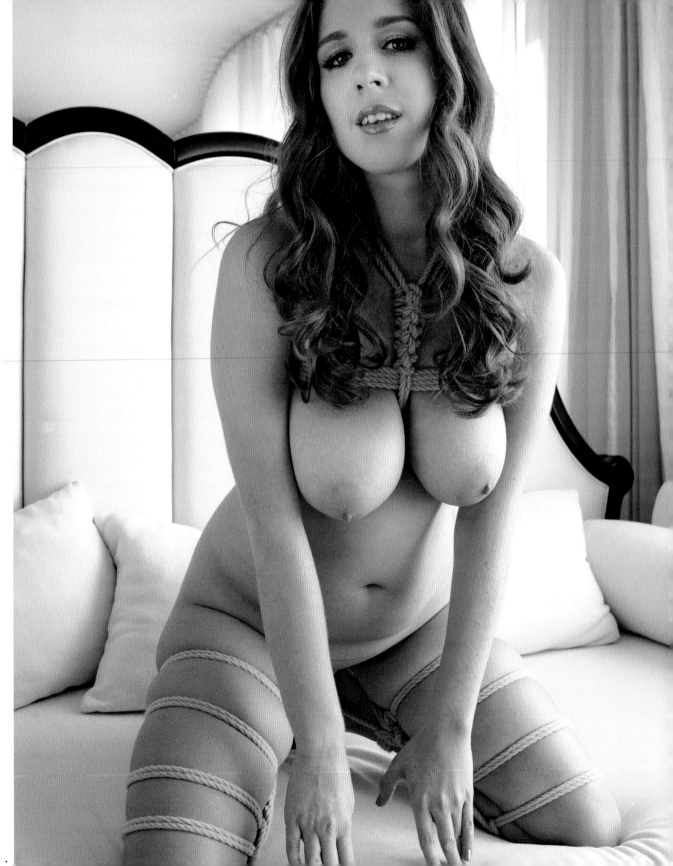

For me, the art and enjoyment starts the moment before the rope falls into place, that specially charged moment where your eyes meet and then your partner's demurely drop and you pull him or her close to you, your hands starting slow, beginning the dance of wrapping and feeling connected to your partner. Of feeling your partner relax and exhale and fall into the dance of binding and caressing. Of your partner's head relaxing back against your chest as you carefully tie him or her, watching your partner forget his or her cares and worries and just be in that moment with you. Where there is nothing but you two, and what you are doing, and the rest of the world falls away. That is what I love most and I hope you have a chance to experience it as well.

FINDING A BDSM COMMUNITY

If you've taken your first steps into bondage with your long-term partner(s), and you've both loved it so much that you want to make it a larger part of your life, then your next step might be finding the bondage/BDSM community in your city. This isn't to imply that you have to go straight from a little light wrist bondage and blindfolding to hardcore swinging—far from it. There are many benefits that being part of a community can give you, and not all of them are orgasm-related (although the best benefits of anything are always orgasm-related, if you ask me). Think of the BDSM community like a book group: You don't sit around reading books with your book group, do you? No; you discuss books, recommend good reads to each other and drink wine while waxing lyrical about the virtues of Jane Austen over the Brontës. In other words, you share in each other's knowledge about a subject that you all enjoy. Your inclusion in a BDSM community can be just the same; meeting likeminded people to share the best places to get colored rope and bondage tape, and which creams help bruising go down to avoid awkward questions.

◄ *This tie uses a very simple Futo, which makes Alex look gorgeous.*

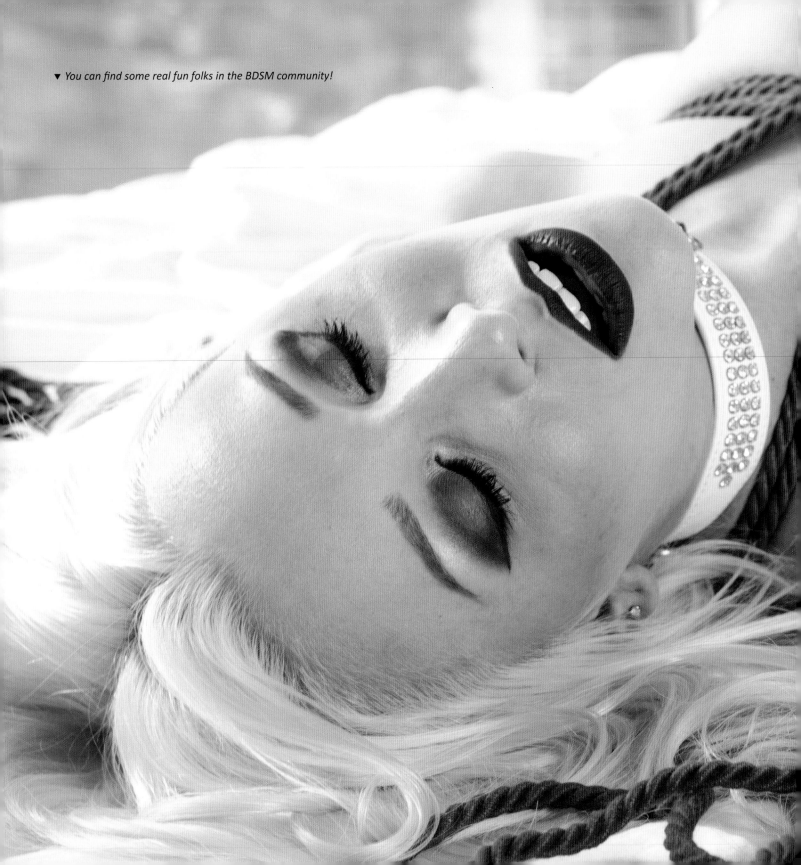
▼ *You can find some real fun folks in the BDSM community!*

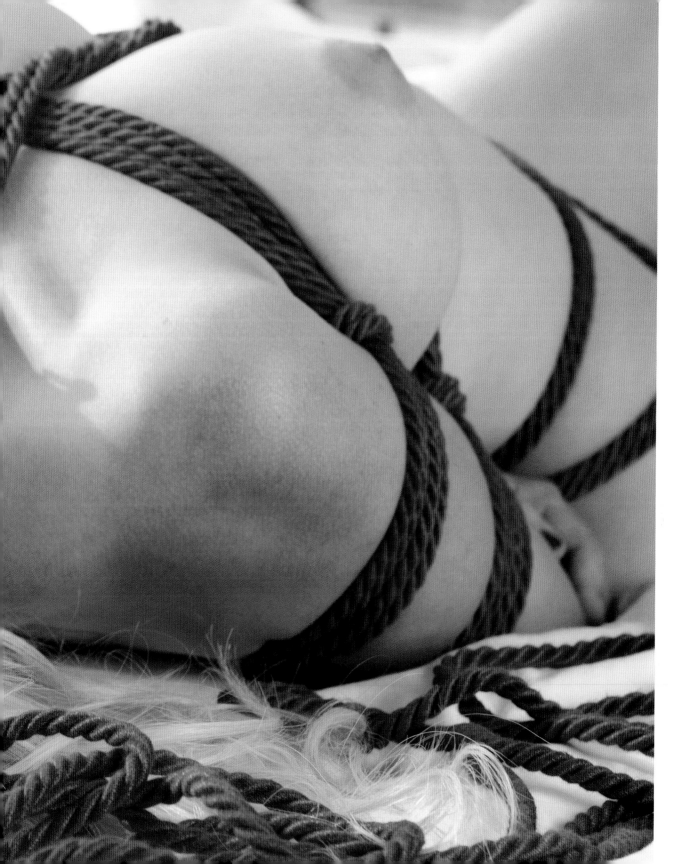

On the other hand, one of you might have coyly mentioned over a chai latte and a cookie that you might, just maybe, once in a while, be interested in bringing someone else into your playtime. Your partner might have shyly agreed that a third (or fourth, or fifth) play friend might be fun also. You might have timidly high-fived about it. In that case, then you might be looking for your local BDSM community in order to meet other likeminded kinksters who just love being tied up and spanked as much as you do. Great! Come in from the cold and pull up a chair; there's a lot here for you!

People anywhere and everywhere love being tied up, so even if you live out in Small Town, Nowhere, you can be sure that someone will share in your hobby—even if it is the old crone who runs the post office. I'll wager that there's a thriving bondage community in every city and large town in North America, although the larger the city you call home, the wider the pond of sexy little fish for you to play with. Of course, it doesn't matter how many there are if you don't know where to find them—so where's the best place to look?

No matter where you are in the world, Fetlife.com is a great resource for finding folks who share your kinky interests (and for looking at some sizzling hot photos). Like a Facebook for the perverted, Fetlife is a social media site made by and for those who love nothing more than being trussed up like a Christmas turkey on a school night. There's a page listing kinky meetups, also known as "munches," by city, and you can also search people by their location. This doesn't mean that you should turn into a Web stalker trying to contact other people—the rules of normal social interaction still apply! If you like the look of someone, send him or her a private message saying a little bit about yourself and your interests, and that you're looking for a community near you. Don't go straight into listing your dirtiest of desires, because then you'll be the internet equivalent of that pervy old man in the brown coat down the street. Always be polite.

Google will also be your friend in your search for frisky friends; simply search "BDSM [your town]" or "bondage [your town]" and you're sure to find dozens of listings of meetups, events, play parties, and even classes in your area. It's important at this point to know what you're looking for. Do you want to enjoy a drink with some friendly people to chat and make friends and, if you see a spark with any of them, maybe take it further? Or do you

The sky's the limit! ▶

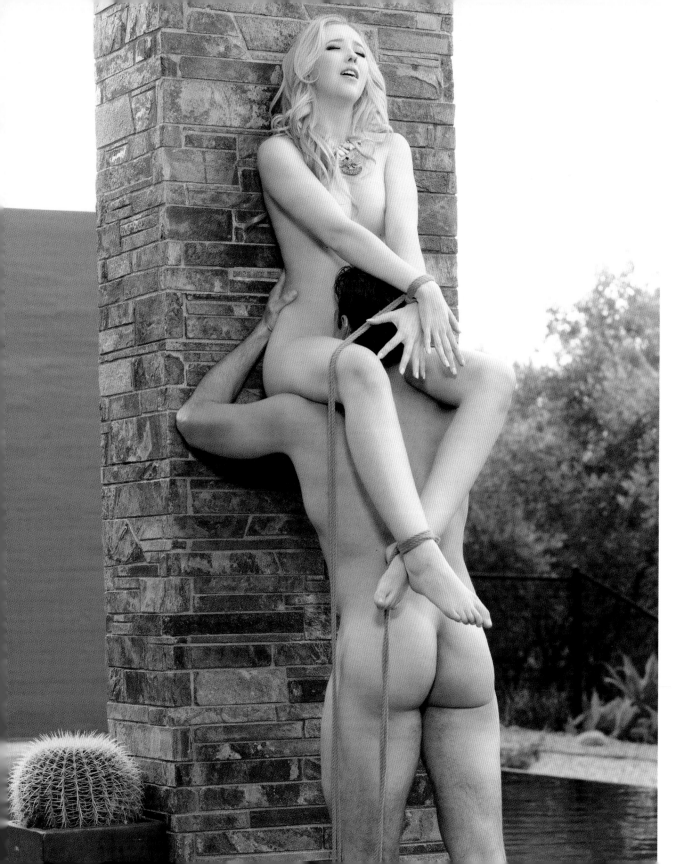

want to dive headfirst into the play party scene, where sex is everywhere and you'll find gorgeous nubiles bound in rope, waiting to be played with? These options and everything in between will most likely be available: Kinksters are generally loud and proud, and they aren't shy about putting themselves out there, so see what's going on where you live and get yourself out to an event. Once you've met one rope-loving friend, you're sure to find many more—and then who knows where the fun will end?

Some people will tell you that they found sexy strangers on Craigslist, and that this turned into one of their most fulfilling bondage/BDSM-based relationships. That's absolutely wonderful for them, but searching Craigslist for sexy, interesting people is like shopping at Target on Black Friday: You might find something wonderful, but you'll have to risk your sanity and your limbs to do so. The anonymity of Craigslist and the ease of posting mean that you can never be sure who's behind the username, so I would recommend proceeding with great caution on that site; at the very least, if you arrange to meet up with someone, go with your friend or partner and make sure that someone knows where you are.

Once you find some people around you who love the same things that you love, and can hold your hand (and anything else you might like held) while you delve deeper into the scene, you'll find yourself in a whole new world of kinky fun time, whether you're on your own or with a partner/partners. There really is nothing like being part of a solid, sexy community full of exciting people and kinky opportunities, and you might find yourself organizing parties, events, and meetups before you know it! Don't be afraid to put yourself out there, as underneath all the latex and leather, the BDSM community is a loving, cuddly place full of wonderful people, and they'll welcome you with open arms (and open legs) no matter who you are.

But don't forget what your mum told you: Never play with strangers.

BRINGING KINK INTO YOUR DAILY LIFE

For some, a semiregular night getting tied up by the wrists and ankles and ravished with numerous sex toys and an almighty amount of lube (water-based if you're using condoms, remember) is more than enough bondage. For others, like me, the realization that life without bondage just isn't as fun comes quickly, and the calendar becomes more and more crowded with nights set aside for evenings full of rope, tape, leg spreaders, and squealing. However, as time-poor individuals with barely enough time to dress and eat before getting the kids to school before work (and the moms in the playground still whisper about that memorable morning when you got so tangled up in breakfasts and packed lunches that you forgot to put on a top), it can be difficult to find a space in your daily life to set aside a little adult playtime.

Some people find that simply fitting bondage or BDSM into a few nights per week, or on their few days off, simply isn't enough. These people crave kink all day long, and yearn for the freedom that they find by operating within set roles. If you can relate to this and you've already spent a good long time in a power exchange relationship, you may find that a 24/7 Total Power Exchange relationship is for you. This is a partnership in which one partner gives up total control of their lives to another, to live as a submissive all day, every day. In this kind of relationship, the lives of both (or all) partners are completely defined by their roles as dominant and submissive; for instance, the submissive will leave all decision making up to the dominant, and they may even express the relationship in public by having the dominant lead the submissive around and make the sub perform tasks for him or her. This is, of course, a very intense type of situation, and most people won't ever feel themselves totally ready for this type of arrangement.

If you don't feel that a full time D/S relationship is what you're looking for, then there are many other ways of ensuring that bondage and discipline are mainstays in your daily life. For instance, if you are mistress and you want your submissive partner to feel your presence all day long, why not have him wear your underwear under his pinstripe suit, so that in meetings with the CEO he can feel the lace of your panties gently tickling his balls, rendering him with a permanent semiboner hidden beneath the desk? Or, if you're a dominant with a naughty submissive who needs to be reminded whom she belongs to, why not gently tie two of her fingers together with red wool and send her off on her day, reminding her whether she's at work, at a bar with friends, or at home in bed that at least a little of her freedom now belongs to you?

Of course, bringing bondage into your routine can be as simple as setting aside an hour before bed to relax and destress with a little rope-based playtime. Step away from the computer or the TV and engage in something that you're truly passionate about and that makes you feel free every time you do it. You don't have to spend hours crafting ornate ties every day. Your practice can be as simple as tying your submissive's hands and feet together and telling him how much you care about him. Bondage can be a force for great good in a relationship, so use it as a way to cement the connection that you feel with your partner. Make bondage the thing that you enjoy alone, with no friends around, no kids knocking at your bedroom door, and no phones ringing all the time.

RESOURCES

ROPE

I believe in supporting small artisans who craft rope exactly to my specifications. Support your local and not-so-local rope makers. Artists need to pay the bills too.

Colored cotton rope: Hand Made Rope, handmaderope.com

Colored bamboo spun rope: Omega Rope, omegarope.com

Natural: Moco Jute, m0cojute.com

Light natural and red: Knotty Kink, knottykink.com/bondage-rope

BOOKS

There are a number of fantastic rope bondage books on the market, as well as a vast array of BDSM books that can help you to explore your sexuality. Hopefully, some of these will help you signpost your journey into kink.

How to be Kinky: A Beginner's Guide to BDSM (2008). Morpheous. Green Candy Press, San Francisco.

How to be Kinkier: More Adventures in Adult Playtime (2010). Morpheous. Green Candy Press, San Francisco.

Two Knotty Boys Showing You the Ropes (2006). Two Knotty Boys. Green Candy Press, San Francisco.

Two Knotty Boys Back on the Ropes (2010). Two Knotty Boys. Green Candy Press, San Francisco.

Erotic Bondage Handbook (2000). Jay Wiseman. Greenery Press, San Francisco.

The Seductive Art of Japanese Rope Bondage (2002). Midori. Greenery Press, San Francisco.

Bondage for Sex (2006). Chanta Rose. BDSM Press.

FASHION

I want to thank my stylist team, Mia and AJ from Apt 9 Productions.

Apt 9 Productions
www.apt9productions.com

Thank you to the Stockroom for their generosity in donating the fetish clothing for the shoot. Boutique located at 2809 ½ W. Sunset Blvd., Los Angeles, CA 90026

The Stockroom
www.thestockroom.com

Thank you to the following clothing manufacturers:

Syren Latex Fashion
www.syren.com

Stormy Leather
www.stormyleather.com

PHOTOGRAPHY

Holly Randall: Thank you to Holly and her team, who shot the majority of this book, including the instructional photos. I am grateful to have had the chance to work with such a perfectionist. hollyrandall.com

Myself: Stand-alone images and cover photo. lordmorpheous.com

Geoff George Photography: I am forever grateful to Geoff for doing my pickup shots at odd hours of the day while the book was racing toward a deadline and I was in the slow lane.

MODELS

Thank you to all the models: Allura, Aaliyah Love, Samantha Rone, Kourtney Kane, Ryan Driller, Celeste Star, Ana Foxx, Spencer Scott, Sophia Jade, Princess, Josie, Marie McCray, Stevie Shae, Alex Chance, Zoey Monroe, Dani Daniels, Selma Sins, and My Allyss.

ABOUT THE AUTHOR

Morpheous is a sex educator, author, photographer, and kinkster based in Toronto. This is his third book, following on the heels of his popular BDSM books *How to be Kinky: A Beginner's Guide to BDSM* and *How to be Kinkier: More Adventures in Adult Playtime* (2008 / 2012, Green Candy Press, San Francisco). Morpheous's work is archived in the Sexual Representation Collection of the University of Toronto's Mark S. Bonham Centre for Sexual Diversity Studies, at the Leather Archives and Museum in Chicago, and at the National Archives of Canada.

Morpheous has taught a variety of workshops on rope bondage, the aesthetics of bondage, fetish photography, advanced and beginner BDSM, and workshops catered to professional dominants and submissives. He travels and presents regularly, doing outreach to both academic and kink-aware safer sex organizations as well as performing in rope bondage expos the world over.

He is also the founder of Morpheous' Bondage Extravaganza, an annual rope bondage art installation that has grown over the years into the world's largest public rope bondage event, broadcasting to bondage fans all over the globe over the internet. Though the event started as a part of Toronto's annual Nuit Blanche all-night art festival, it has recently expanded to include another MBE night in Orlando, Florida. mbeworldwide.com.

You can find out more about Morpheous at lordmorpheous.com.

ACKNOWLEDGMENTS

A very special thank you goes to my team of riggers, Allura, Ruairidh, and Ve-ra, without whose artistic skills this book would not be filled with the myriad of beautiful images of rope bondage art that grace the pages.

Allura is a passionate rigger hailing from Toronto, Ontario, and has been practicing rope seriously for two years. She first encountered rope bondage and suspension at Subspace fetish parties and was immediately taken by its beauty and practicality. Through events like Rope Bite and Shibaricon, along with studying others' rope on the internet, her skill and passion flourished. She is heavily influenced by Milla Reika, Ve-ra, and tons of local Toronto riggers, as well as little ol' me. She practices rope bondage one to two hours a day and is a firm believer in the healing power of rope.

Ruairidh (pronounced *roo-ah-ree*) is a Toronto-born-and-bred rope artist who's been interested in bondage since he could tie his own shoes. Over the years, he has developed a distinctive style of rope weaving, covering bodies with large-scale rope creations that range from beautifully severe bondage to severely beautiful fashion apparel. Ruairidh draws inspiration for his art from a wide array of sources including nature, old architecture, modern engineering, and even haute couture. He has been teaching weaving techniques for several years at his local bondage groups and Shibaricon. Find Ruairidh at ruairidh.ca or on Fetlife.

Ve-ra first discovered her fascination with bondage at an art festival, and since then has had the privilege of working with some of the world's best talent in this arena. Inspired mostly by ballet and contemporary dance, she has used her knowledge of the physical body to create works of art with Japanese-influenced rope. Since having first gotten lessons through her local community, she has been able to meet and learn from talented rope artists such as Wykd Dave and Clover, Peter Slemrian, Yukimura Haruki, and, most recently, Kazami Ranki. Ve-ra now teaches rope bondage internationally, sharing her love of rope with anyone with the passion to learn the art, and I've been lucky enough to come along on her journey too.

INDEX

ALSO AVAILABLE FROM QUIVER

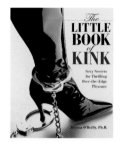

The Little Book of Kink
978-1-59233-574-9

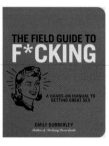

The Field Guide to F*cking
978-1-59233-509-1

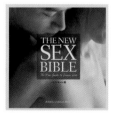

The New Sex Bible
978-1-59233-603-6

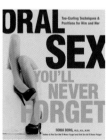

Oral Sex You'll Never Forget
978-1-59233-593-0